# PLANT-BASED
# AND DAIRY-FREE
# COOKBOOK

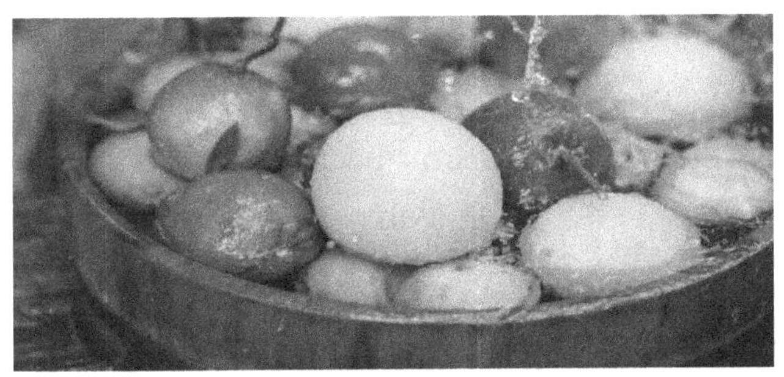

## Easy and Nutritious
## Recipes to Maintain a
## Clean and Healthy Eating
## Diet

**Terri Hogan**

# TABLE OF CONTENTS

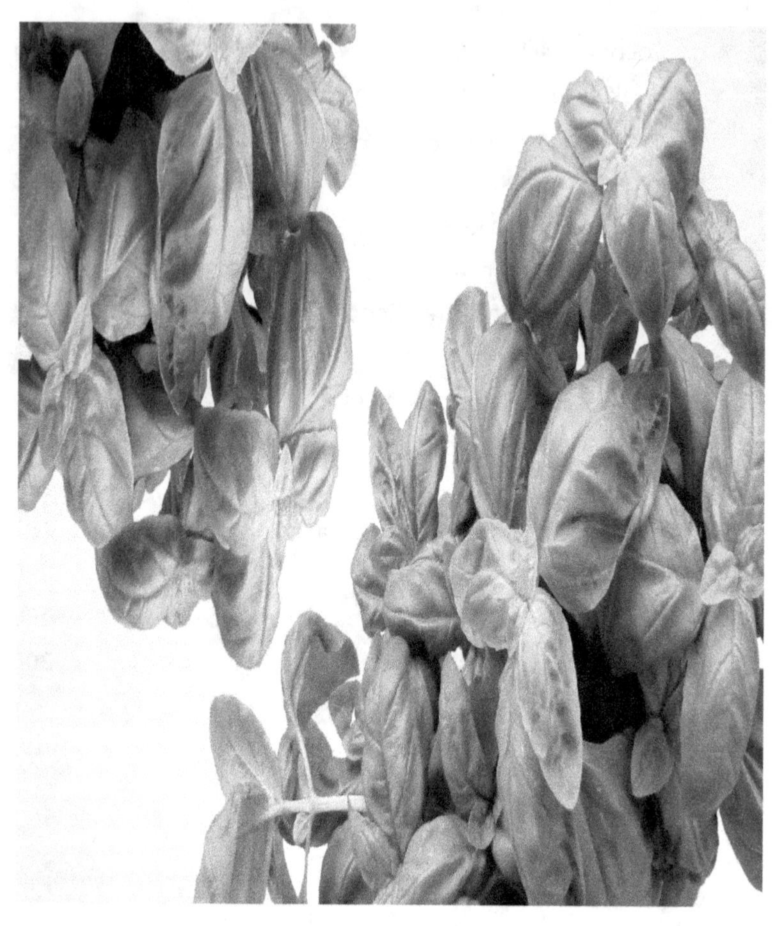

# INTRODUCTION

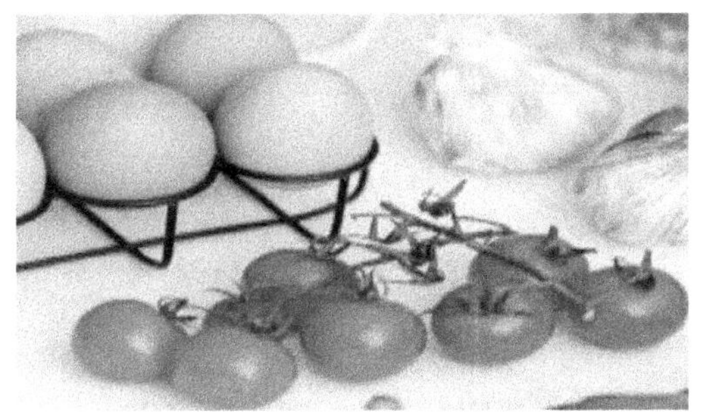

In the heart of a bustling city, where culinary adventures unfold, a revolution in the kitchen is quietly taking root. Enter the world of the "Plant-Based Diary-Free Cookbook," a masterpiece designed for those seeking a vibrant and healthful journey into the realm of plant-based, dairy-free cuisine.

Meet Terri Hogan, a culinary enthusiast on a mission to redefine the way we nourish ourselves. The cookbook unfolds with her story, a tale of rediscovery and transformation through the tantalizing flavors of plant-derived wonders. As she embarks on this wholesome adventure, she shares her culinary secrets, unveiling a symphony of colors and tastes that elevate every meal to a masterpiece. From energizing breakfasts that greet the day with vitality to sumptuous dinners that soothe the soul, each recipe in the "Plant-Based Diary

Free Cookbook" is a celebration of the earth's bounty. Discover the art of crafting delectable dishes without dairy, where almond milk and coconut cream reign supreme, and where the harmonious blend of vegetables, legumes, and grains dances on the palate.

This cookbook is not just a collection of recipes; it's an invitation to a lifestyle that harmonizes with the rhythm of nature. Join Terri Hogan on a culinary odyssey, where every page tells a story of mindful, compassionate, and flavorful living. In the pages of "Plant-Based Dairy-Free Cookbook," the kitchen becomes a sanctuary, and each meal is an

expression of love for the self and
the planet.

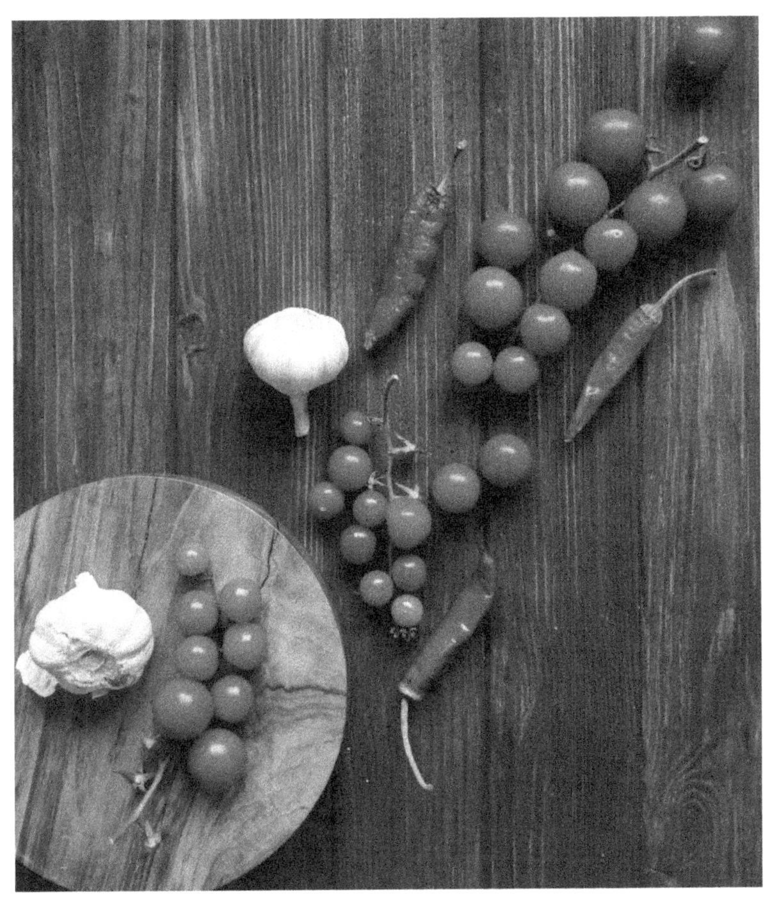

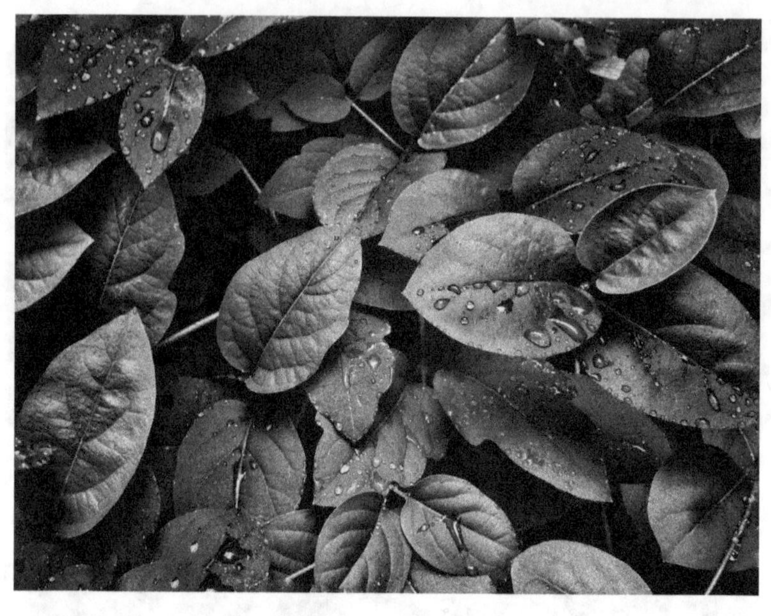

# CHAPTER ONE

## What does Plant-Based and Diary-Free eating mean?

A plant-based and dairy-free diet is a dietary approach that promotes plant-derived foods while avoiding or limiting the use of animal products, notably dairy. Here's an explanation of each term:

## Plant-Based Eating Plan:

A plant-based diet consists of whole, plant- derived foods such as fruits, vegetables, legumes, grains, nuts, and seeds. It restricts or prohibits the intake of animal products such as meat, dairy, eggs, and honey. The emphasis is on obtaining the majority of nutritional requirements from plant sources.

## Dairy-Free Eating Plan:

A dairy-free diet eliminates all dairy products, including milk, cheese, butter, yogurt, and other cow's milk products. This restriction is frequently caused by lactose intolerance, a milk allergy, ethical considerations, or as part of a plant-based diet.

People adopting a plant-based and dairy-free diet seek to derive their nutrients, proteins, and fats primarily from plant sources, ensuring a diverse and well-balanced intake. Common alternatives to dairy products in this lifestyle include plant-based milk options (almond milk, soy milk, coconut
milk, etc.), non-dairy cheeses, vegan butter, and plant-based yogurts.

This dietary choice is often associated with health benefits, environmental sustainability, and ethical considerations related to animal welfare. It's essential for individuals on such a diet to plan meals thoughtfully to ensure they meet their nutritional needs, including essential vitamins and minerals that may be more concentrated in animal products.
Consulting with a healthcare professional or nutritionist can provide personalized guidance for those

considering or adopting a plant-based, dairy-free diet.

# CHAPTER TWO

## Benefits of Plant-Based and Diary-Free eating

Plant-based and Dairy-free eating can offer various benefits, including:

1. **Improved Heart Health:** Plant-based diets are associated with lower risks of heart disease due to reduced intake of saturated fats and cholesterol found in animal products.

2. **Weight Management:** Plant-based diets
are often rich in fiber, promoting a feeling of fullness and aiding in weight management.

3. **Better Digestive Health:** A plant-based diet typically includes a variety of fruits, vegetables, and whole grains, contributing to a healthier digestive system.

4. **Reduced Cancer Risk:** Some studies suggest that plant-based diets may lower the risk of certain cancers, possibly due to the abundance of antioxidants and phytochemicals in plant foods.

**5.Environmental Sustainability:** Plant- based diets tend to have a lower environmental impact, as they generally require fewer resources like water and land compared to animal agriculture.

6. **Ethical Considerations:** Choosing plant- based and dairy-free options aligns with ethical considerations for many people, as it reduces reliance on animal products and supports more humane treatment of animals.

7.**Better Blood Sugar Control:** Plant-based Diets may help improve insulin sensitivity and regulate blood sugar levels, reducing the risk of type 2 diabetes.

8.**Reduced Inflammation:** Some individuals experience reduced inflammation on a plant-based diet, which may alleviate symptoms of inflammatory conditions.

It's important to note that individual

responses to dietary choices can vary, and it's advisable to consult with a healthcare professional or a nutritionist to ensure a balanced and adequate nutrient intake.

# CHAPTER THREE

## Essential ingredients for plant based diary free cooking

In the vibrant world of plant-based, dairy- free cooking, a palette of essential ingredients awaits, transforming ordinary dishes into culinary masterpieces. At the heart of this gastronomic revolution lies the rich diversity of fruits, vegetables, grains, nuts, and seeds, each offering a unique contribution to flavor, texture, and nutrition.

First and foremost, plant-based cooking thrives on the abundance of fresh produce — from crisp leafy greens to jewel-toned berries and succulent, ripe tomatoes. These ingredients not only infuse meals with vibrant colors but also provide an array of vitamins, minerals, and antioxidants essential for vitality.

Whole grains such as quinoa, brown rice, and oats become the cornerstone of hearty plant-based meals, offering a satisfying foundation packed with fiber and complex carbohydrates. Legumes, including chickpeas, lentils, and black beans, bring a protein-packed punch, elevating dishes to new heights of nutritional excellence.

Navigating the plant-based pantry, almond milk, coconut cream, and cashew butter emerge as dairy-free champions, imparting creamy textures and decadent richness. Meanwhile, flaxseeds, chia seeds, and hemp seeds add a nutritional boost, enhancing meals with omega-3 fatty acids, fiber, and plant-based protein.

In the realm of plant-based, dairy-free cooking, these essential ingredients serve as the building blocks of a culinary symphony where innovation and nourishment dance in perfect harmony, creating a feast for the senses and a celebration of wholesome living.

## Frozen Edamame beans

Edamame, also known as soy beans, is high in protein, iron, and calcium, which help carry oxygen to muscles and

strengthen bones. They're also high in gut-friendly fiber, with half a cup supplying nearly a fifth of your daily fiber requirements. They're
vibrant, green, and crunchy, and they're great for adding color and protein to grain or bean salads.

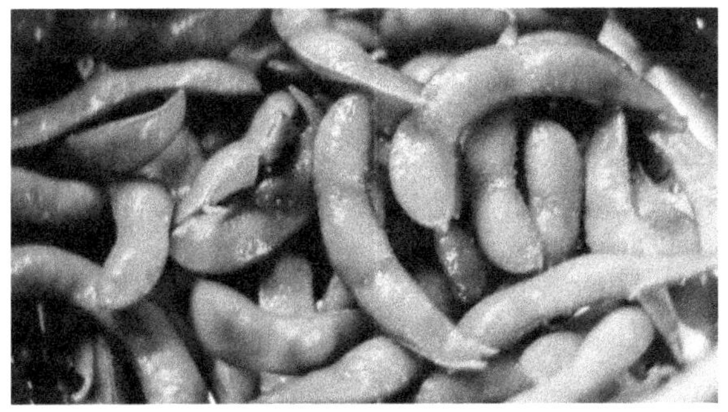

## Lentils

Canned lentils are a convenient and flexible item that will boost the fiber and protein content of any meal. Dried lentils cook rapidly and, unlike most legumes, do not require pre-soaking. Both varieties contribute to your five-a-day requirement. Combine dried versions with soups and stews.

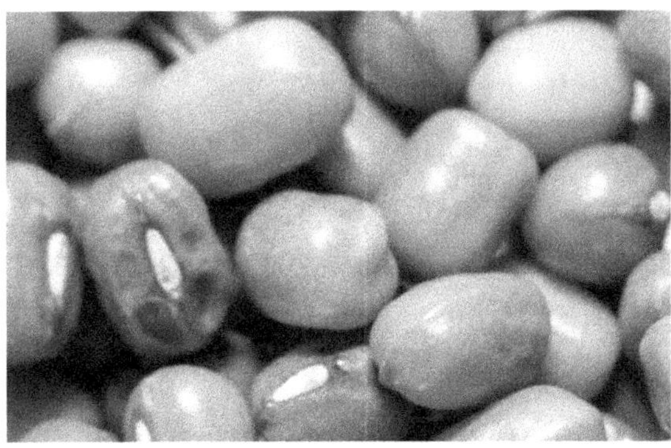

## Canned Beans

It's worth keeping a few cans of beans on hand because they're so versatile and high in protein, carbs, and fiber. Choose those that have been canned in water with no additional salt. You may use them to make burgers, dips, and hummus in addition to your favorite bean salads.

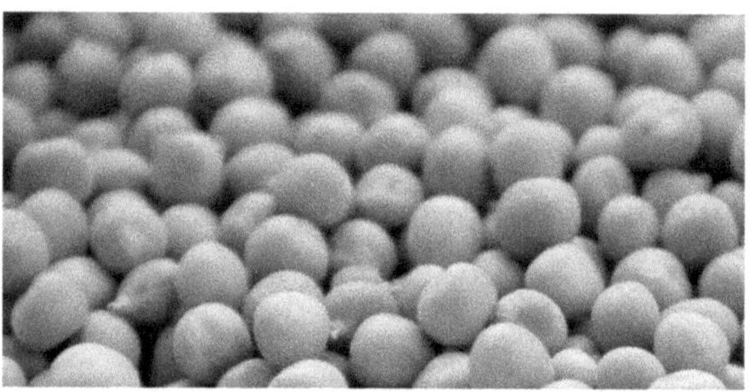

## Tempeh

Protein and vitamins abound in this fermented soy bean cake. Before throwing into salads and stir-fries, or stuffing pitas, bake with a spicy marinade. Tempeh is more nutritious than tofu, with more than double the protein and much more B vitamins.

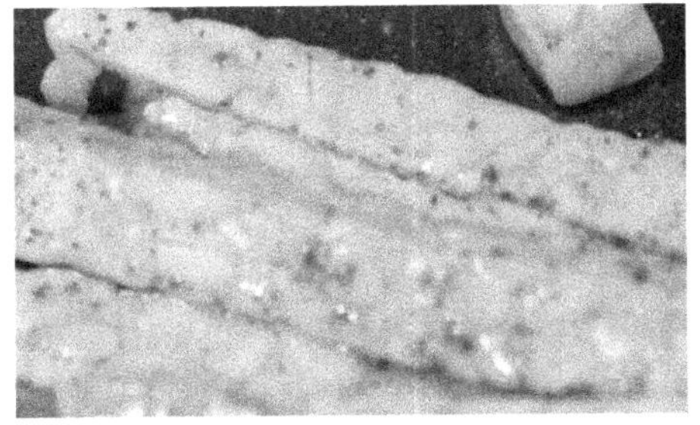

## Quinoa

Ouinoa includes all of the essential amino acids and is high in protein and carbohydrates. Buy dried to cook from scratch or in ready-to-heat pouches when time is of the essence. Use rice or pasta in soups and salads.

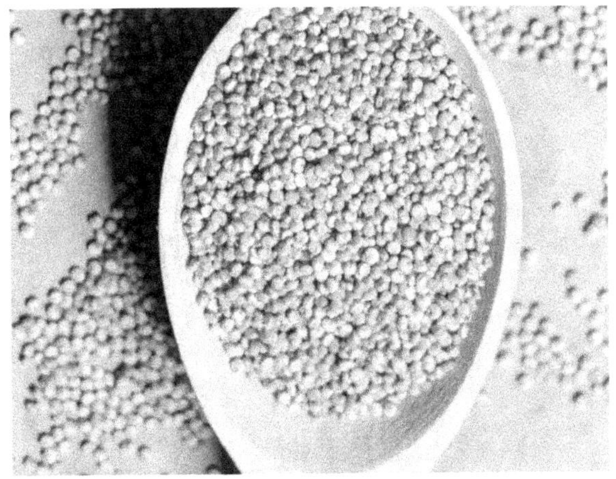

**Tofu**

Tofu is derived from soy and can be firm or silky. Tofu with a firm texture is commonly used in kebabs, curries, and stir-fries. The silken version has a silky texture, making it ideal for healthy cheesecakes and smoothies. Plain tofu absorbs seasonings and other flavors effectively, making it suitable for

both savory and sweet meals. A 125g piece of tofu contains half the calories of a grilled chicken breast while providing a quarter of the woman's daily protein.

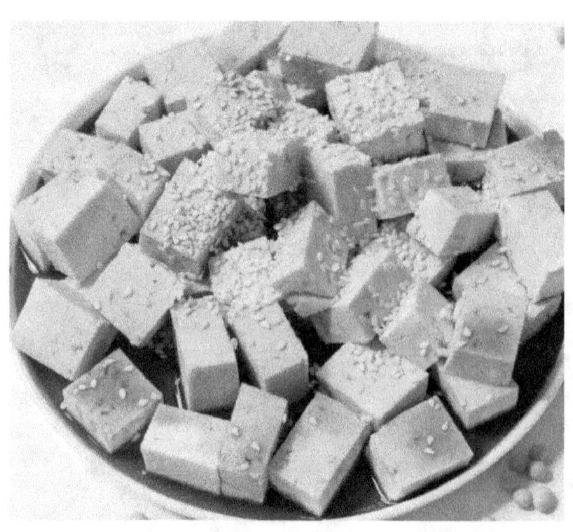

## Eggs

They're an important, protein-rich quick snack that's also high in minerals like zinc and vitamin B. Boil, scramble, whisk into omelettes, or use leftover vegetables to make fritters or frittata.

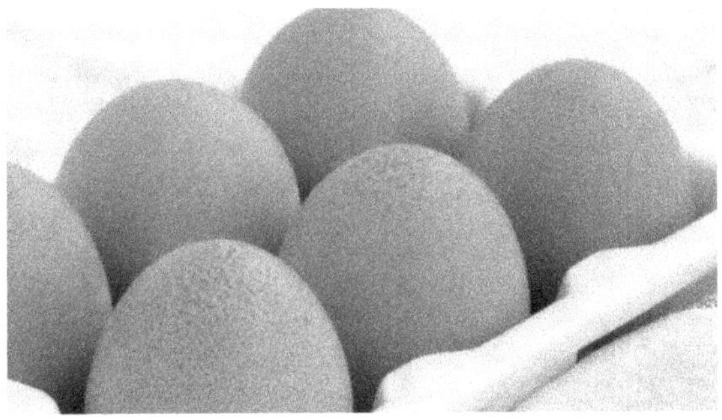

## Frozen peas

Peas can enhance almost any recipe because they're so flexible! With roughly 5g of protein per 100g, they can make a significant impact in your protein (as well as your five-a-day) intake.

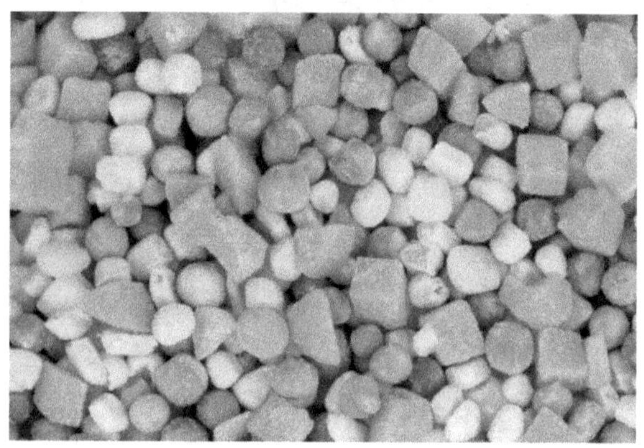

# CHAPTER FOUR

## Breakfast Delights

### Vegan Pancakes:

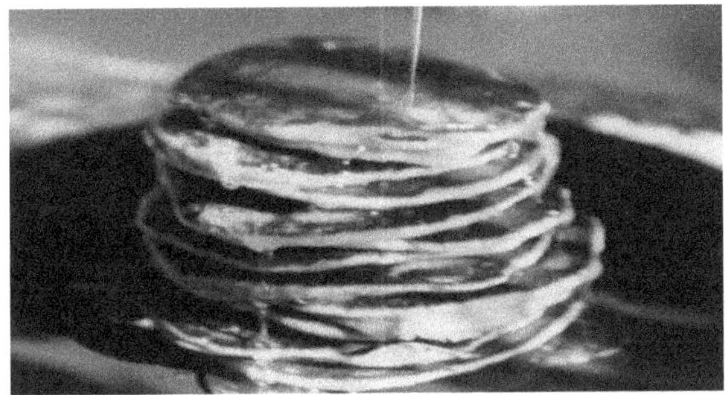

The basic recipe below can be used to make vegan pancakes.

### Ingredients:

- One cup of ordinary flour
- One teaspoon sugar
- Two tsp. of baking powder
- One teaspoon of salt
- One cup nondairy milk (oat, soy, or almond milk

are the best options)
- Vegetable oil, two tablespoons
- one teaspoon vanilla extract

**Guidelines:**

1. In a mixing bowl, whisk together flour, sugar, baking powder, and salt.
2. In a separate bowl, mix the vegan milk, vegetable oil, and vanilla extract.
3. Mix the wet ingredients with the dry ones just enough to barely combine them. Don't overmix; a few lumps should be acceptable.
4. Heat a griddle or nonstick skillet over medium heat.
5. Spoon 1/4 cup of batter onto the pan for each pancake.
6. Cook until surface bubbles appear, then turn and continue cooking until golden brown on the other side.
7. Continue until the batter is all used. You are welcome to add chocolate chips.
8. Slice bananas or blueberries to

your vegan pancakes. Serve with
your preferred fruit compote or
syrup.

# Chia Seed Pudding

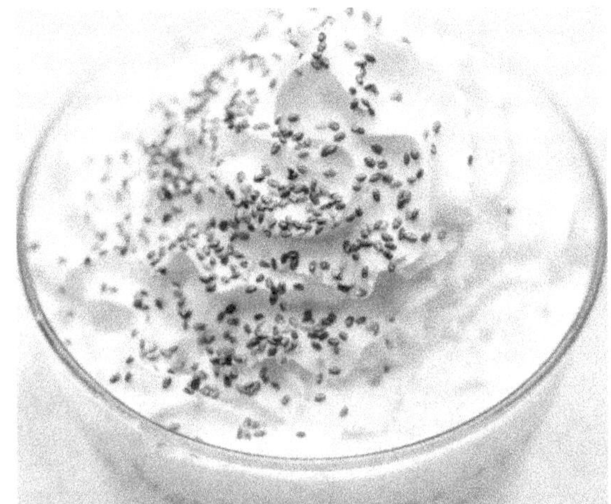

To make chia seed pudding, mix 1/4 cup of chia seeds with 1 cup of your choice of milk (almond, coconut, etc.). Add sweeteners like honey or maple syrup to taste, and stir well. Let it sit in the fridge for at least a few hours or overnight, stirring occasionally until it thickens. Top with fruits or nuts before serving.

# Tofu Scramble

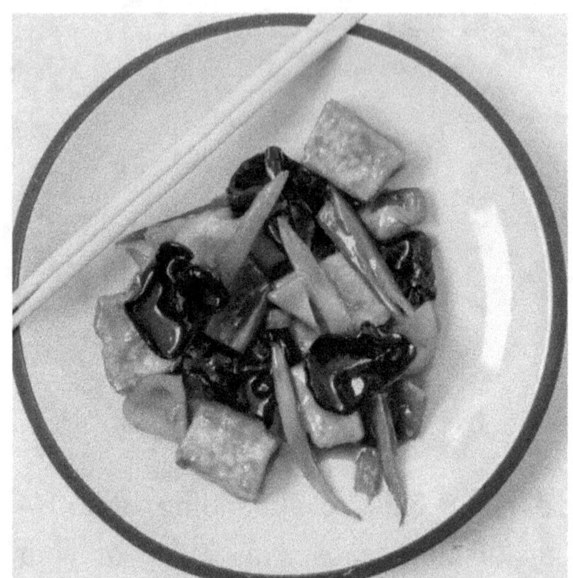

To make tofu scramble, crumble firm tofu in a pan and sauté with veggies like bell peppers, onions, and spinach. Season with turmeric, black salt, pepper, and any desired spices. Cook until heated through and serve as a tasty, vegan alternative to scrambled eggs.

# Avocado Toast with Tomato Salsa

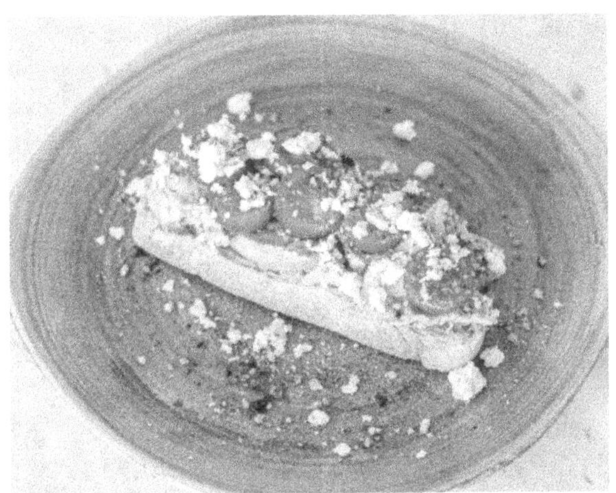

A tasty, wholesome, and easy-to-make food is avocado toast with tomato salsa. For you, here's a simple recipe:

**Ingredients**:

- ☐ Two pieces of whole-grain bread, or any other bread you want
- ☐ One mature avocado
- ☐ One chopped medium-sized tomato
- ☐ 1/4 red onion, chopped finely
- ☐ half a lime, squeezed

☐ Chop some fresh cilantro (optional).

☐ To taste, add salt and pepper.

☐ Optional red pepper flakes for extra spiciness

**Guidelines**

1.  Toast the bread: Toast the bread slices
        until they have the crispiness you like.

2.  Get the avocado ready: Halve the
    avocado and scoop out the pit
    while the bread is browning.
    Empty the flesh of the avocado
    into a bowl.

3.  Mash the Avocado: To get the
    desired amount of creaminess,
    mash the avocado with a fork.
    Season to taste with a touch of
    salt and pepper.

4.  How to Make Tomato Salsa: Place the
    chopped red onion, diced tomatoes, and
    fresh cilantro (if using in another
    bowl). Drizzle the blend with the
    lime juice. Season with salt and
    pepper. Mix
    the ingredients until thoroughly blended.

5. Put Together the Avocado Toast: Over

the slices of toasted bread, equally
distribute the mashed avocado.

5. Put some tomato salsa on top: Drizzle a
liberal amount of tomato salsa over the
mashed   avocado.   Ascertain
that  the  tomatoes  and  onions
are distributed equally.

6. Season and garnish: Sprinkle a bit more salt and pepper over the tomato salsa. If you enjoy a bit of heat, add red pepper flakes for some spice.

7. 0ptional Garnish: Garnish with additional cilantro, lime wedges, or a drizzle of balsamic glaze if desired.

8. Serve Immediately: Avocado Toast with Tomato Salsa is best enjoyed immediately while the toast is still warm and the flavors are fresh.

This Avocado Toast with Tomato Salsa is not only delicious but also packed with healthy fats, vitamins, and minerals. It makes for a satisfying breakfast or snack, offering a perfect balance of creaminess, acidity, and crunch. Feel free to customize the recipe with additional toppings or seasonings to suit your taste preferences.

# Oatmeal with Fruit

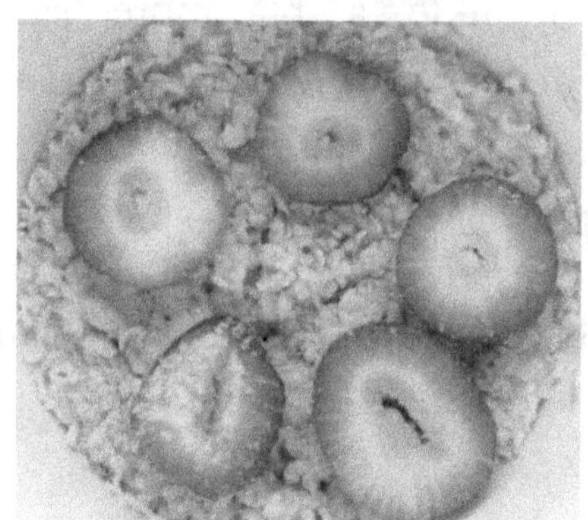

Making oatmeal with fruit is a nutritious and delicious way to start your day. Here's a basic recipe that you can customize with your favorite fruits and toppings:

## Ingredients:

- ☐ 1 cup rolled oats
- ☐ 2 cups water or plant-based milk (almond milk, soy milk, etc.)
- ☐ Pinch of salt
- ☐ 1 ripe banana, mashed
- ☐ 1/2 cup berries (e.g., strawberries, blueberries, raspberries)
- ☐ 1/4 cup chopped fruits (e.g., apple, pear, mango)

- ☐ 1 tablespoon maple syrup or sweetener of choice (optional)
- ☐ Nuts, seeds, or granola for topping (optional)

## Instructions

1.    Cook the Oats: In a saucepan, combine the rolled oats, water or plant-based
milk, and a pinch of salt. Bring to a boil over medium heat.

2. Simmer: Reduce the heat to low and simmer the oats, stirring occasionally, until they reach your desired consistency. This usually takes about 5-7
minutes.

3. Mash the Banana: While the oats are cooking, mash the ripe banana in a bowl.

4. Add Mashed Banana: When the oats are almost done, add the mashed banana to the saucepan. Stir well to incorporate the banana into the oats.

Prepare the Fruit: Wash and chop your choice of fruits. Berries work well, and adding some chopped apple, pear, or mango can add sweetness and texture.

Combine with Oats: Stir the chopped

6. fruits into the cooked oatmeal. The heat of the oats will slightly soften the fruits.

Add sweetness (optional): If you'd like,

7. mix in some maple syrup or other

sweetener of your choice with the oatmeal. To taste, adjust the sweetness.

8.    Serve:Fill dishes with oats and fruit.It can also be moved to a serving platter.

9. Top with Extra Candy(Optional): Granola, almonds, or seeds can be sprinkled over top for extra crunch and
nutrition.

10.    Enjoy:Serve the warm oatmeal with fruit, and savor a hearty and aromatic morning.

Feel free to use your imagination when selecting fruits and toppings to give your oatmeal a special taste. Because of its adaptability, you may modify this recipe to fit your tastes and use the fruits that are in season.

# Coconut Yoghurt Parfait

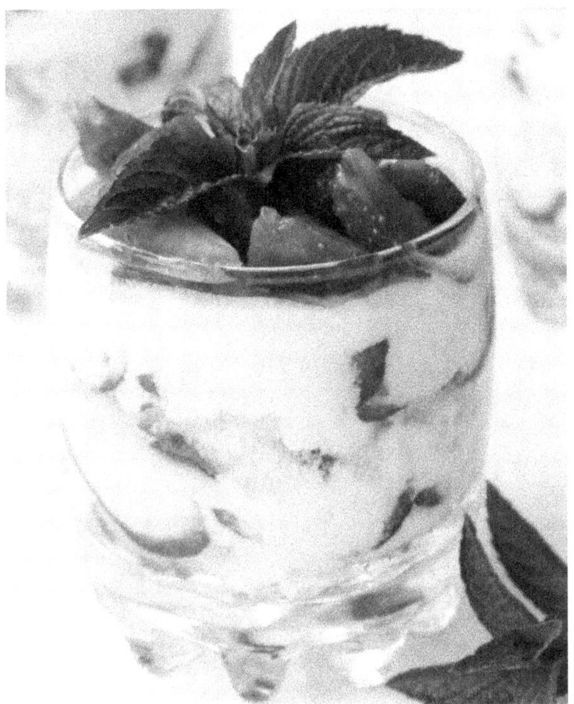

Creating a Coconut Yogurt Parfait is a delicious and refreshing way to enjoy a plant-based, dairy-free treat. Here's a simple recipe for a Coconut Yogurt Parfait:

Ingredients:

- ☐ 1 cup dairy-free coconut yogurt
- ☐ 1 cup mixed berries (strawberries, blueberries, raspberries)

☐  1/2  cup  granola  (choose  a
dairy-free and preferably low-sugar
option)

2 tablespoons shredded coconut 1 tablespoon chia seeds (optional)
Drizzle of maple syrup or agave syrup (optional)

Instructions:

1. Prepare the Coconut Yogurt: If you're not using store-bought coconut yogurt, you can make your own by mixing coconut milk with a vegan yogurt starter or using a store-bought dairy-free coconut yogurt.

   Assemble the Parfait Layers: Start by
2. Spooning a layer of coconut yogurt into the bottom of serving glasses or bowls. Include Berries: Place a layer of mixed

3. berries over the yoghurt. Use frozen berries that have thawed or fresh berries.

   Distribute the Granola: Top the berries

4.  with a coating of granola. This
    gives your parfait more texture and
    crunch.

    Repetition of Layers: Add more berries, a

5.  dollop of coconut yogurt, and a
    layer of granola to repeat the
    layers. Keep
    going until you get to the top
    of the bowl or serving glass.

6.     Addshreddedcoconutontop
:Topthe parfait with shredded
coconut to finish it off. This
intensifies the flavor of the
coconut and gives it a tropical touch.

7. Supplementary:ChiaSeeds:Chiaseeds
can be sprinkled on top or in between
the layers for extra nutrition and texture.

8. DrizzlewithSyrup(Optional):Ifyou
desire additional sweetness, drizzle a bit
of maple syrup or agave syrup over the
tool

5.     ServeImmediately:CoconutYo
gurt Parfait is best enjoyed
immediately while the granola
is still crunchy. If
you're making it ahead of time, you can
refrigerate it and add the granola just
before serving.

6.     Enjoy: Grab a spoon and
enjoy the layers of creamy
coconut yogurt, juicy
berries, and crunchy granolain every
bite.

Feel free to get creative with the

ingredients and customize your parfait with your
favorite fruits, nuts, or seeds. The Coconut Yogurt Parfait is a versatile and delightful dessert or breakfast option that's not only delicious but also packed with plant-based goodness.

# Vegan Overnight Oats:

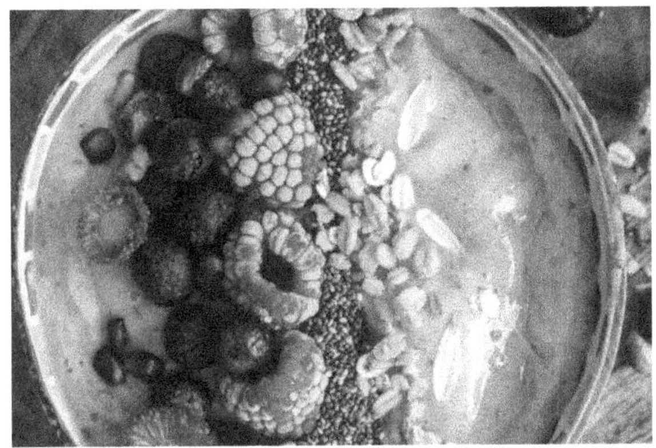

Making Vegan Overnight Oats is a simple and convenient way to enjoy a nutritious and delicious breakfast without any cooking involved. Here's a basic recipe for you to try:

Ingredients:

- 1/2 cup rolled oats
- 1/2 cup plant-based milk (almond milk, soy milk, coconut milk, etc.)
- 1/2 ripe banana, mashed (optional for natural sweetness)
- 1 tablespoon chia seeds
- 1/2teaspoon vanilla extract
- Toppings of your choice: fresh fruit, nuts, seeds, nut butter, or sweeteners like maple

syrup or agave syrup

Instructions:

1. Choose Your Container: Select a jar or a container with a lid that can hold at least one cup of liquid.

2. Combine Ingredients: In the jar, combine the rolled oats, plant-based milk, mashed banana (if using), chia seeds, and vanilla extract.

3. Blend Well: To guarantee that the oats and chia seeds are distributed equally, thoroughly stir the ingredients.

4. Keep Cold All Night: Put the jar in the refrigerator after covering it with a lid.
   Allow the mixture to steep for four to six hours, or overnight. This enables the liquid to seep into the oats and chia seeds, causing them to soften.

Mix Well Before Serving: Mix

5. everything well in the mixture and toss again in the morning. To get the right consistency, thin it out with a splash of plant-based milk if it's too thick.

- Include toppings: Add your own toppings to personalize your vegan overnight oats. Popular options include fresh fruit, nuts, seeds, and a dash of sugar.

7.	PresentandSavor:Youmay eatVegan Overnight Oats right out of the container. You may just grab a spoon and enjoy the delicacy without having to cook.

8.	ExtraAdviceatYour0ption:Tr yout many plant-based milk alternatives to see which flavor you like.

9. Tosuityourtaste,youcanadd additional mashed banana or sweeteners to change the sweetness.

10.	Experimentwithdifferenttas te combinations by adding spices such as nutmeg, cinnamon, or a dollop of nut butter.

Not only are vegan overnight oats delicious, but they're also a handy breakfast alternative that you can customize to your tastes. Go wild with your topping selections and savor a filling and healthy lunch.

# Quinoa Breakfast Bowl

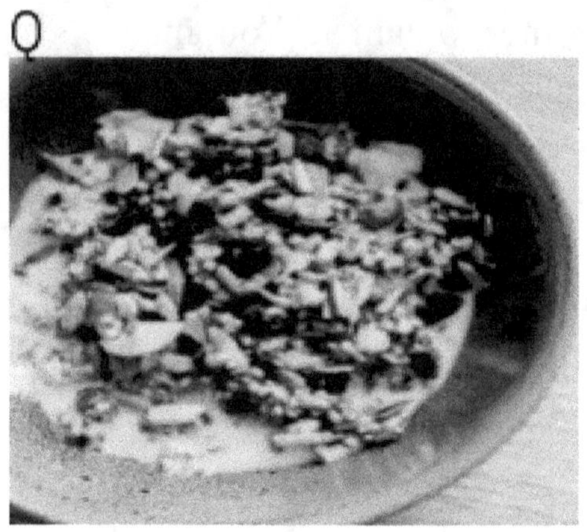

Creating a Quinoa Breakfast Bowl is a nutritious and versatile way to start your day. Here's a basic recipe for a delicious Quinoa Breakfast Bowl.

Ingredients:

- ☐ 1/2 cup quinoa (uncooked)
- ☐ 1 cup plant-based milk (almond milk, soy milk, etc.)
- ☐ 1 ripe banana, sliced
- ☐ 1/2 cup berries (strawberries, blueberries, raspberries)
- ☐ 1 tablespoon nut butter (almond

butter, peanut butter, etc.)

- ☐ 1 tablespoon chia seeds
- ☐ 1 tablespoon chopped nuts (walnuts, almonds, etc.)
- ☐ Optional sweetener: maple syrup, agave syrup, or honey (to taste)

Optional toppings: sliced fruit, coconut flakes, seeds (chia seeds, flaxseeds), or a dollop of yogurt

Instructions:

1.  Rinse Quinoa: Rinse the quinoa under cold water to remove any bitterness.

2.  Prepare Quinoa: Place the washed quinoa and plant-based milk in a saucepan. After bringing it to a boil, lower the heat so that it simmers. Cook, covered, until the quinoa is cooked and the liquid is absorbed, about 15 minutes. Using a fork, fluff the quinoa.

3.  Put the Bowl Together: After cooking, ladle the quinoa into a bowl.

4.  Add berries and sliced banana: Add your preferred berries and sliced
bananas on the top of the quinoa.

5. Pour over some Nut Butter: Pour some nut butter on top of the fruit and quinoa.
   Almond butter, peanut butter, or any other nut butter of your choosing can be used.

6. Add chopped nuts and chia seeds: For more texture and nutrition, top the bowl
   with chopped nuts and chia seeds.

7. OptionalSweetener:Ifyouprefer
additional sweetness, drizzle with
maple syrup, agave syrup, or honey
according
to your taste.

8.     OptionalToppings:Addany
additional toppings you like,
such as sliced fruit,
coconut flakes, or a dollop of
plant- based yogurt.

9.     MixandEnjoy:Gentlymixa
llthe ingredients in the bowl.
Your Quinoa Breakfast Bowl is
ready to be enjoyed!

This breakfast bowl is highly customizable, so feel free to experiment with different fruits, nuts, and toppings to suit your taste preferences. Whether you enjoy it warm or cold, this Quinoa Breakfast Bowl provides a hearty and nutritious start to your day.

# Chickpea Flour Pancakes

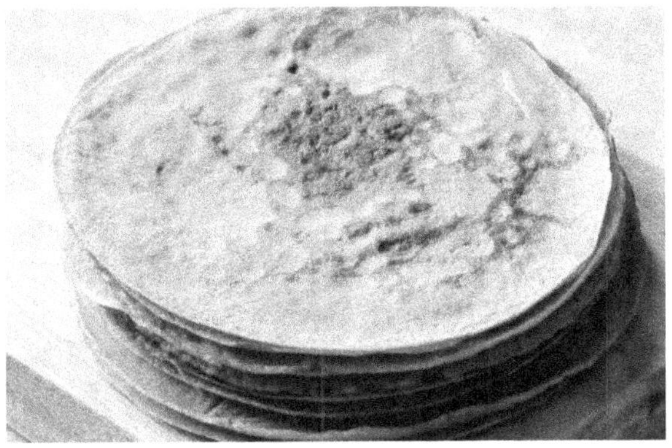

Chickpea flour pancakes, also known as besan or gram flour pancakes, are a tasty gluten-free alternative to regular pancakes. Here's a basic recipe for Chickpea Flour Pancakes:

Ingredients:

- 1 cup chickpea flour (besan/gram flour) ☐ 1 cup water 1/2 teaspoon baking powder ☐ 1/2 teaspoon turmeric powder (optional, for color)
- 1/2 teaspoon cumin powder
- 1/2 teaspoon coriander powder
- 1/4teaspoon black salt (kala namak) or ordinary salt
- 1/4teaspoon black pepper (optional)

□ 1/4 cup finely chopped onions (optional) □ 1/4 cup chopped tomatoes (optional)

1/4 cup chopped cilantro (optional) Greasing the pan with cookingoil or ghee

Instructions:

1. Combine the dry ingredients: In a mixing bowl, combine chickpea flour, baking powder, turmeric powder (if using), cumin powder, coriander powder, salt, and black pepper.

2. Pour in the water: To avoid lumps, gradually add water to the dry ingredients while mixing. Continue whisking until the batter is smooth. The batter should have the consistency of regular pancake batter.

3. Optional vegetable additions: To add flavor and texture, finely chopped onions, tomatoes, and cilantro can be added to the batter.

4. Allow the Batter to Rest: Allow

at least 15-20 minutes for the batter
to rest. This aids the absorption of
the chickpea flour
and improves the texture of the
pancakes.

Preheat the pan as follows: Over

5.

medium heat, heat a nonstick or well-

greased skillet or griddle.

6.    Pourthebatter:Whenthepani
sheated, add a ladle of batter into
the center and spread it out into a
thin, circular shape.

7. Cookthepancake:Cookthepancake
    for two to three minutes on one
side, or until bubbles form on the
surface and
the edges begin to lift.

8. Turnoverandcook:0ncethepanca
    ke has turned golden brown on
    all sides,
    fry it for a further one to two
minutes on the other side.

9.    Again:Proceedwiththelefto
verbatter, lightly oiling the pan
before each pancake.

10. Warm Serving: Warm chickpea
    flour pancakes should be
    served. They go nicely with
    yogurt, chutney, or any
other topping you like.

Not only are these Chickpea Flour

Pancakes tasty, but they are also free of gluten and packed with protein. To suit your tastes, feel free to experiment with the batter by adding your preferred herbs, spices, or veggies.

# Sweet Potato Breakfast Hash

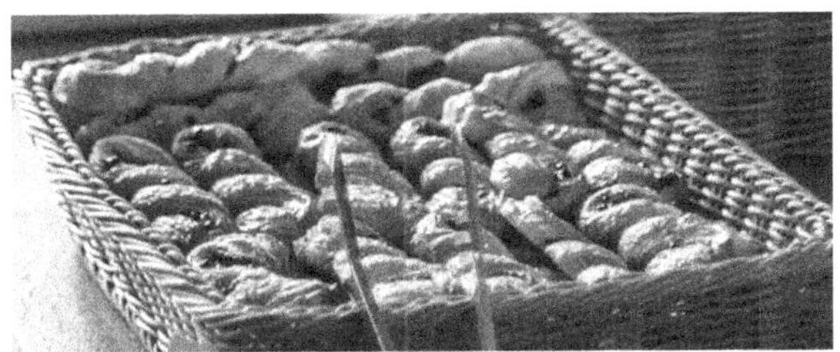

Sweet potatoes, veggies, and spices come together in this tasty and filling recipe to make a satisfying breakfast hash. A basic recipe for Sweet Potato Breakfast Hash can be found here:

Ingredients:

- ☐ Peel and dice two medium-sized sweet potatoes.
- ☐ One sliced bell pepper of any color
- ☐ One finely chopped red onion, two minced garlic cloves, one cup cherry tomatoes, cut in half, and one cup chopped spinach or kale
- ☐ One tsp of paprika
- ☐ Half a teaspoon of cumin

Half a teaspoon of chili powder, or to taste

Add salt and pepper to taste. Use two tablespoons of cooking oil (such as avocado or olive oil).

Extra toppings at your discretion: chopped cilantro, avocado slices, and fried or poached eggs

Guidelines:

1. Get the sweet potatoes ready: Sweet potatoes should be peeled and chopped into bite-sized bits.

2. Sauté Vegetables: Heat the cooking oil in a large skillet or frying pan over medium heat. Add the diced sweet potatoes and cook for about 5-7 minutes, stirring occasionally until they start to soften.

3. Add Onions and Garlic: Add the chopped red onion and minced garlic to the skillet. Continue to cook for another 3-5 minutes until the onions are translucent and the sweet potatoes

are tender.

4. Add Bell Pepper: Add the diced bell pepper to the skillet and cook for an

additional3-4 minutes until the pepper begins to soften.

5.      SeasonwithSpices:Sprinkle the paprika, cumin, chili powder, salt, and pepper over the vegetables. Stir well to
coat the sweet potatoes and veggies with the spices.

6.   Addthegreensandtomatoes:Addthe chopped kale or spinach and cherry tomato halves. Simmer for a further two
to three minutes, or until the leaves are wilted and the tomatoes are starting to gO soft.

7.      Modifytheseasoning:1fnecessary, taste the hash and adjust the seasoning. Depending on your taste, you can add extra spices, salt, or pepper.

8.      Serve:AftertheSweetPotato Breakfast Hash is cooked through and seasoned, serve it on plates.

9.      Add-ontoppings:Addoptiona

ltoppings to each serving, such as chopped cilantro, avocado slices, or fried or poached eggs.

10.	SavorWarm:Warmupthisdi shof sweet potato breakfast hash and enjoy the wonderful blend of tastes and textures.

This Sweet Potato Breakfast Hash is not only a tasty and satisfying breakfast but also a versatile dish that you can customize with your favorite vegetables and toppings. It's a great way to start the day with a nourishing and hearty meal.

## Vegan French Toast

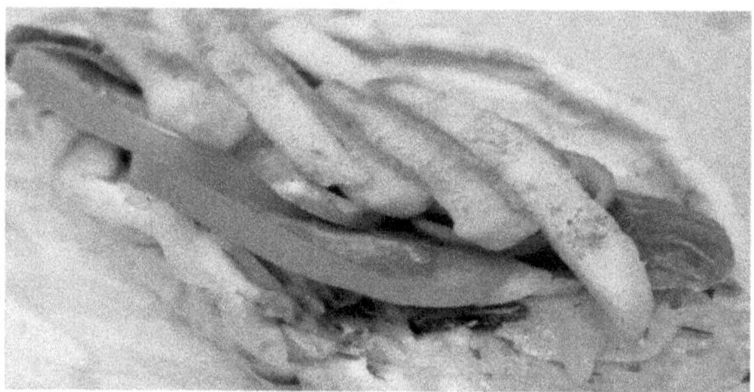

Certainly! Making Vegan French Toast is easy and delicious. Here's a simple recipe for you:

Ingredients:

4 slices of your favorite vegan bread (such as whole wheat or sourdough)

1 cup plant-based milk (almond milk, soy milk, oat milk, etc.)

2 tablespoons chickpea flour (also known as besan or gram flour)

1 tablespoon nutritional yeast (optional, for a slightly cheesy flavor)

1 tablespoon maple syrup or agave syrup

1 teaspoon ground cinnamon O 1/2 teaspoon vanilla extract O A pinch of salt

O Coconut oil or vegan butter for frying O Optional toppings: fresh fruit, maple syrup, powdered sugar

Instructions:

1. Get the batter ready: Mix the plant- based milk, peanut flour, nutritional yeast (if using, maple syrup, ground cinnamon, vanilla essence, and a small amount of salt in a shallow dish. Make care to thoroughly mix the batter.

2.  Let the Bread Soak: Make sure both sides of each bread slice are coated by dipping them into the batter. Give the bread a brief period of time to soak up the mixture.

3.  Warm Up the Pan: Over medium heat, preheat a skillet or nonstick pan. Coat

the pan with a little quantity of vegan butter or coconut oil.

4. MaketheFrenchtoast:Thebr eadslices should be soaked and cooked for two to three minutes on each side, or until they are golden brown and beginning to crisp up.

5. Repeat:Continuewithther emaining slices of bread.

6.KeepWarm:0ncecooked,keepthe French toast warm in a low oven while you finish the remainder of the meal.

7. Serve:WarmVeganFrenchT oastwith your favorite toppings. Fresh fruit, maple syrup, or powdered sugar are all good additions.

8. Enjoy:Enjoyyourtasty,cr uelty-free Vegan French Toast!

Feel free to get creative with your toppings and to try with different bread types. This recipe offers a vegan alternative to regular French toast that is just as fulfilling and delectable.

# Vegan Breakfast Burrito Bowl

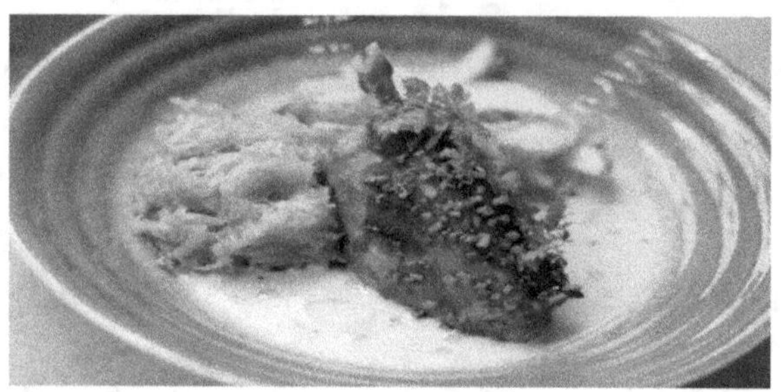

Creating a Vegan Breakfast Burrito Bowl is a flavorful and satisfying way to start your day. Here's a simple recipe for you:

Ingredients:

For the Bowl:

B 1cupcookedquinoaorbrownrice
B
1cupblackbeans,drainedandrinsed (canned or cooked)
B
1cupsautéedtofuortempeh,dice
d B 1cupcookedcornkernels
B 1avocado,sliced
B
Freshsalsa(store-boughtorhomemade)
B Freshcilantro,chopped
B Limewedgesforgarnish

For the Tofu Scramble:

B
1blockfirmtofu,pressedandcrumbled
B 1tablespoonoliveoil
B
1/2onion,finelychopp
ed                              B
1bellpepper,diced

☐   2 cloves garlic, minced

☐   1 teaspoon ground cumin

☐   1/2 teaspoon turmeric (for color) ☐      Salt and pepper to taste


Instructions:

To make the Tofu Scramble, follow these steps:

1. Warmtheoliveoilinapanover
     medium heat. Sauté the onions and bell peppers until tender.

     2.      Totheskillet,addthemincedgarl icand crumbled tofu. Cook for 5-7 minutes, or until the tofu is well heated and slightly
browned.

3.   Seasonwithcumin,turmeric,salt,and pepper to taste. To blend, stir everything together thoroughly. Set aside after
removing from the heat.

4.   PreparetheBowl:Layerthecook

ed quinoa or brown rice as the basis in serving bowls.

5.  Ontopofthegrains,layerblackbeans, sautéed tofu or tempeh, and cooked corn.

6. On one side of the bowl, layer sliced avocado and a large tablespoon of fresh salsa.

7. GarnishandServe:Sprinklechopped cilantro over the bowl and garnish with
lime wedges.

8. OptionalAdditions:Customizeyour bowl with additional toppings such as
   vegan cheese, hot sauce, or a drizzle of tahini.

9. MixBeforeEating:Before eating,mix the ingredients in the bowl to distribute
flavors evenly.

10. Enjoy: Your Vegan Breakfast Burrito Bowl is ready to enjoy! Dig in and savor the delicious combination of
flavors.

Feel free to customize the ingredients based on your preferences, and this bowl can be a versatile and nutrient-packed breakfast option.

# Fruit Salad with Almond Yogurt

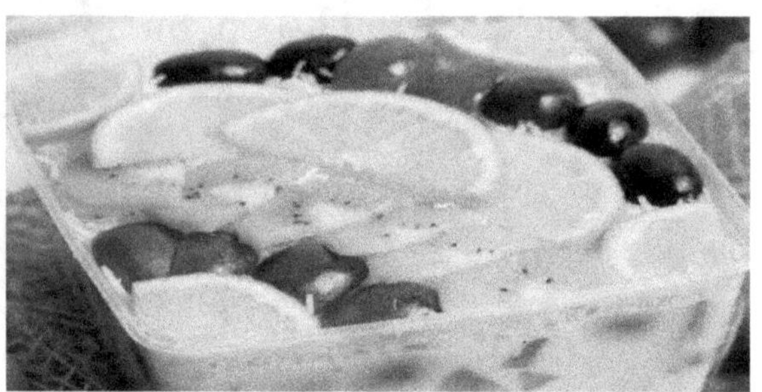

Creating a Fruit Salad with Almond Yogurt is a refreshing and healthy option for a light breakfast or snack. Here's a simple recipe for you:

Ingredients:

To make the Fruit Salad:

B
2cupsmixedfreshfruits(berries,melon, grapes, kiwi, pineapple, and so on)
B  1tablespoonchoppedfreshmintleaves (optional, for garnish)

Dressing with Almond Yogurt:

B
1cupalmondyogurt(purchased or homemade)

B
1to2tablespoonsmaplesyruporaga
ve syrup (to taste)
B atspvanillaextract

1 tablespoon almond slices
(optional, for decoration)

Instructions:

1. Make the Fruit: Wash and cut up fresh fruits into bite-sized pieces. For a visually pleasing salad, combine colors and textures.

2. To prepare the Almond Yogurt Dressing: In a mixing dish, combine the almond yogurt, maple syrup or agave syrup, and vanilla extract. To taste, adjust the sweetness.

3. Assemble the Fruit Salad: In a large mixing bowl, combine the mixed fresh fruits. Gently toss them together to mix.

4. Add the Almond Yogurt Dressing: Pour the almond yogurt dressing over the
fruit salad. Use a spatula or spoon to gently fold the

dressing into the fruit until evenly coated.

5. Chill (Optional): If time allows, you can refrigerate the fruit salad for about 15-
30 minutes to let the flavors meld and the salad cool slightly.

6. Garnish:Sprinklechoppedfreshmint
       leaves over the fruit salad for a burst of
       freshness. If desired, add almond slices
on top for a crunchy texture.

7.      Serve:Spoonthefruitsaladin
toserving bowls or plates.

8.    Enjoy:Drizzlealittlemorealmo
       nd yogurt dressing over each
       serving if
desired, and enjoy your delicious
Fruit Salad with Almond Yogurt!

This fruit salad is not only a
delightful treat for your taste buds but
also a nutritious and hydrating option.
Feel free to customize the fruit
selection based on what's in season or
your personal preferences.

# CHAPTER FIVE

## Lunch          and          Dinner
## Creations

## Lentil Soup

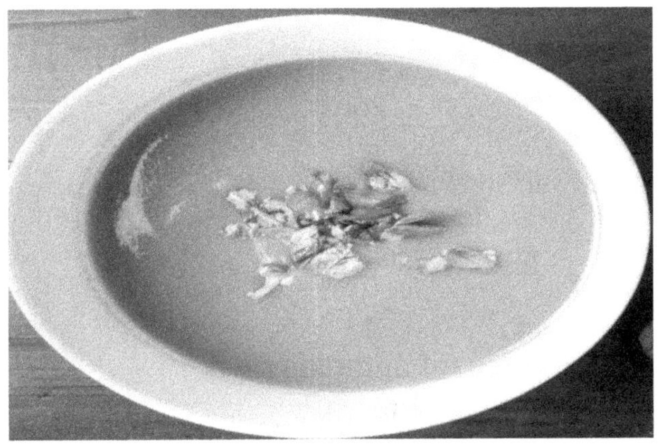

To make a simple lentil soup:

Ingredients:

- ☐ 1 cup dried lentils (rinsed and drained)
- ☐ 1 onion (diced)
- ☐ 2 carrots (chopped)
- ☐ 2 celery stalks (chopped) ☐ 2 cloves garlic (minced)

1 can diced
tomatoes 6 cups
vegetable broth
1 teaspoon ground cumin
1 teaspoon ground
coriander Salt and pepper
to taste Olive oil for
sautéing

Instructions:

1. In a large pot, sauté onion,
   carrots, celery, and garlic in
   olive oil until softened.
2  Add lentils, diced tomatoes,
   vegetable broth, cumin, coriander,
   salt, and pepper. Bring to a boil,
   then reduce heat and simmer for
   about 25-30 minutes or until
3  lentils are tender.
4  Adjust seasoning to taste.
   Optional: blend a portion of the soup for a
5  creamier consistency.
   Serve hot, garnished with fresh herbs or

a squeeze of lemon if desired.

¿    Enjoy your hearty lentil soup!

7

# Quinoa Salad

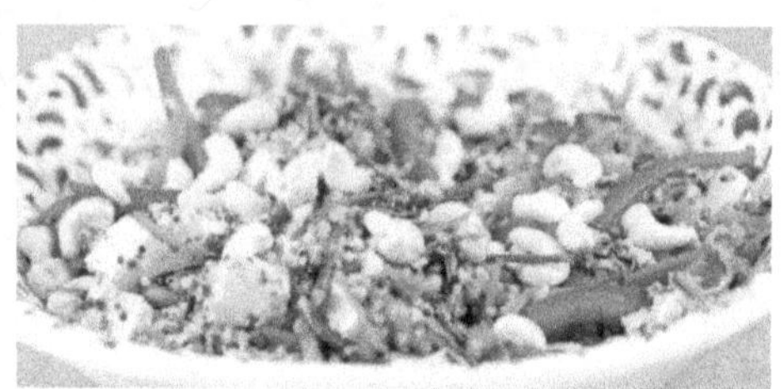

For a delicious quinoa salad:


Ingredients

- ☐ 1 cup quinoa (rinsed)
- ☐ 2 cups water or vegetable broth ☐ Cherry tomatoes (halved)
- ☐ Cucumber (diced)
- ☐ Red bell pepper (diced)
- ☐ Red onion (finely chopped) ☐ Fresh parsley (chopped)
- ☐ Feta cheese (crumbled, optional) ☐ Olive oil
- ☐ Lemon juice
- ☐ Salt and pepper to taste

Guidelines:

1. Wash the quinoa in cool water. Quinoa should be combined with broth or water in a saucepan. After bringing to a boil, lower heat, cover, and simmer the quinoa for fifteen minutes, or until it is tender and the water has been absorbed. Let it cool.

2. Cool quinoa, cherry tomatoes, cucumber, red onion, red bell pepper, and parsley should all be combined in a big bowl.

3. Mix the olive oil, lemon juice, salt, and pepper in a small bowl. To suit your taste, adjust.

4. After adding the dressing to the quinoa mixture, toss to fully incorporate.

5. Add some crumbled feta cheese, if using.

To bring out the flavors, let it sit in the

6. fridge for at least half an hour before serving.

7. Savor this healthy and energizing quinoa salad!

# Stir-Fried Mushrooms

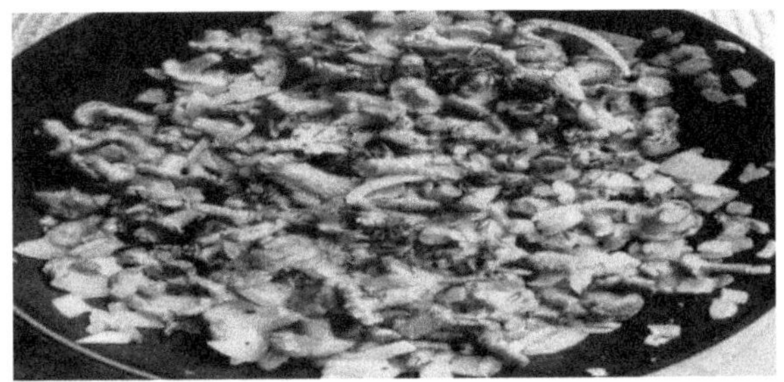

To make a delicious stir-fried mushroom:

Ingredients list:

- ☐ Two cups sliced mushrooms
- ☐ One onion and one bell pepper, cut into slices
- ☐ minced garlic cloves, two
- ☐ a single spoonful of soy sauce
- ☐ One tablespoon of oyster sauce (more taste optional)
- ☐ A single spoonful of vegetable oil ☐ A tsp of sesame oil
- ☐ (Chopped, for garnish) green onions
- ☐ (Optional, as a garnish) sesame seeds

Guidelines:

1  In a wok or big skillet over medium- high heat, heat the vegetable oil.
Stir-fry the sliced mushrooms for two to three minutes, or until they begin to

2  color.

3.  Stir in the onion and bell pepper slices. After the vegetables are crisp-tender, stir-fry them for a further two to three minutes.

4  Stir the minced garlic for around 30 seconds until it becomes aromatic. Over the vegetables, drizzle soy sauce and oyster sauce. Stir to ensure even

5  coating.

6  For added flavor, drizzle some sesame oil over the stir fry.
Cook for a further one to two minutes, making sure that everything is

7  thoroughly cooked and combined.

8.

9.

10.

Add sesame seeds and sliced green
onions as garnish.
Serve the stir-fried mushrooms with
noodles or rice.
Savor your tasty and speedy stir-fried
mushrooms!

# Chickpea and Vegetable Stir- Fry

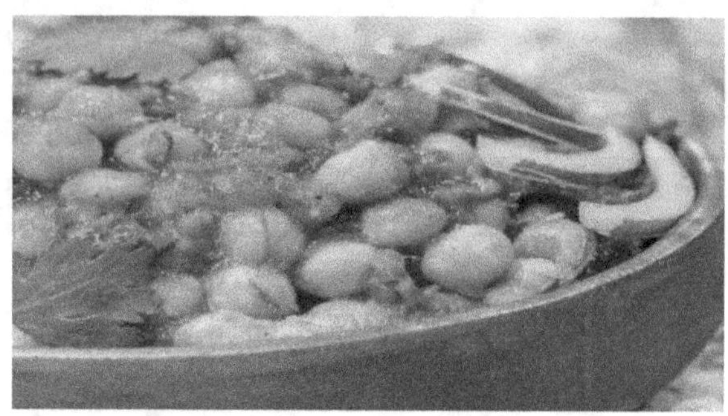

This recipe is simple to make, satisfies hunger, and is full of nutrients. I'll give you a basic recipe here:

Ingredients:

1.5 cupscooked chickpeas,or1 can (15 oz) of rinsed and drained chickpeas

Two cups of chopped mixed veggies (carrots, broccoli, bell peppers, snap peas, etc.)

☐ One finely sliced onion

☐ two minced garlic cloves

One tablespoon of grated ginger

Two tablespoons tamari or soy sauce (for a gluten-free version)
One tsp of hoisin sauce

One tablespoon of sesame oil

One tablespoon of cooking-grade vegetable oil
One teaspoon of optionally spicy chili garlic sauce or sriracha
Add optional garnish of green onions and sesame seeds.
Ready-to-serve cooked rice or noodles

Guidelines

1. Get the chickpeas ready: Pour out and wash the canned chickpeas. Follow the directions on the package to prepare and drain the dry chickpeas if using them.

2 Assemble the Sauce: Combine

the sriracha (if using), sesame
oil, hoisin sauce, and soy sauce
or tamari in a small bowl.
Remove from the way.

3. Add the vegetables and stir-fry: On medium-high heat, heat the vegetable oil in a big skillet or wok. Chopped garlic, grated ginger, and sliced onions should be added. Until aromatic, stir-fry for one to two minutes.

4. For a further three to five minutes, or until the mixed veggies are crisp-tender, add them to the skillet and stir-fry.

5. Put Chickpeas Here: When the veggies in the skillet are ready, add the chickpeas. Heat well while stirring to mix.

6. Add the Sauce: Over the mixture of veggies and chickpeas, drizzle the prepared sauce. To uniformly coat everything, give it a good stir.

7.  Complete and Add a Garnish: Simmer
    for a further two to three minutes, or
    until the sauce starts to thicken and
    the food is well cooked. Taste and
    adjust the seasoning.

8.  As a garnish, top the stir-fry with
    chopped green onions and sesame
    seeds, if using.

9. Serve:Servethestir-friedchic kpeasand vegetables over noodles or cooked rice.

10. Enjoy:Savoryourtastyandnouri shing stir-fried chickpeas and vegetables!

You can change the amount of spice or add your own vegetables to this recipe to make it your own. This is a very adaptable dish that makes a healthy and satisfying evening supper.

# Spaghetti with Vegan Bolognese

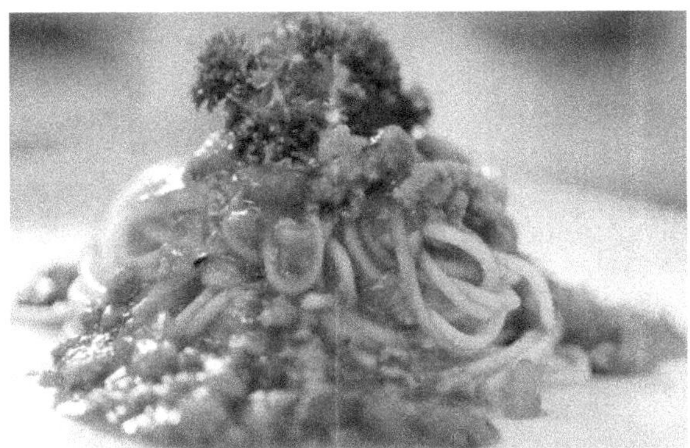

Making Spaghetti with Vegan Bolognese is a flavorful and satisfying plant-based alternative to the classic meat-based dish. Here's a simple recipe for you:

Ingredients:

For the Vegan Bolognese:

B 1tablespoonoliveoil

B 1onion,finelychopped

B 2carrots,peeledanddiced
B 2celerystalks,diced
B 3clovesgarlic,minced

B

    1can(15oz)lentils,drainedandr insed (or cooked green or brown lentils)

B 1can(14oz)crushedtomato es B 2tablespoonstomatopaste
B 1teaspoondriedoregan o B 1teaspoondriedbasil
B 1/2teaspoondriedthyme

B 1bayleaf
B Saltandpeppertotaste

B 1/2cupredwine(optional)

B

1/2cupvegetablebroth

For the Spaghetti:

B

12oz(340g)spaghetti(oryourfavorit
e pasta)

B Saltforboilingwater

B

Garnishwithfreshparsleyorbasil,i
f desired.

B

0ptionalveganParmesancheese
garnish

Guidelines:

1.  Get the vegan Bolognese ready: In a
    big pot or deep skillet, warm up the
    olive
    oil over medium heat. Add the
    chopped celery, carrots, and
    onions. Vegetables should be

sautéed for five to seven minutes to soften them.

2   Add the minced garlic and cook, stirring, for one to two more minutes, or until fragrant.

3.  Add the crushed tomatoes, tomato paste, bay leaf, salt, pepper, dried thyme, dried basil, and dried oregano.
MiX
thoroughly to blend.

4.  Pour the drained lentils into the pot and stir well.

5.  Pour the red wine (if using} into the saucepan and simmer it for a few minutes to reduce the alcohol content.

After adding the veggie broth and stirring, heat the mixture to a simmer. Simmer, covered, over low heat for at least half an hour, stirring now and then. It will get more tasty the longer it simmers.

7.  Prepare the spaghetti: Heat salted water in a big pot until it boils. Cook the pasta until al dente, following the directions
on the package.

8. Put Together and Serve: Take off the bay leaf from the Bolognese vegan sauce.

9. Over the cooked pasta, pour the Bolognese sauce.

10. If preferred, garnish with vegan Parmesan cheese and fresh basil or
parsley.

11.    Enjoy: Savor this tasty vegan Bolognese with spaghetti!

12. With its robust flavor profile, this vegan Bolognese sauce is ideal served over
your preferred pasta.

13. Adjusttheseasoningstosuityourtaste,
and feel free to add extra vegetables or herbs if you like.

# Mushroom and Spinach Stuffed Bell Peppers

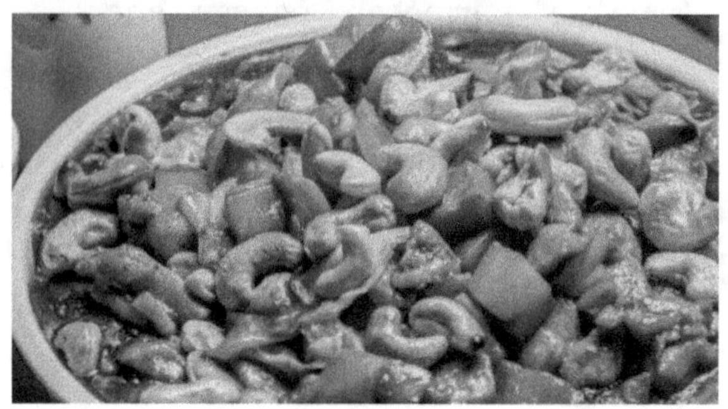

Making Mushroom and Spinach Stuffed Bell Peppers is a delicious and nutritious option for a satisfying meal. Here's a simple recipe for you:

Ingredients:

4 large bell peppers (any color) 1 tablespoon olive oil

1 onion, finely chopped

2 cloves garlic, minced

8 oz (about 225g) mushrooms, finely chopped

2 cups fresh spinach, chopped

1 cup cooked quinoa or
rice 1 teaspoon dried
thyme Salt and pepper,
to taste

1 can (15 oz) black beans, drained
and rinsed

1 cup tomato sauce or marinara sauce

1 cup vegan cheese, shredded (optional)

Fresh parsley or cilantro for garnish
(optional)

Guidelines:

1.  Set the oven to preheat: Warm up your
    oven to 375°F, or 190°C.

2       Arrange the bell peppers: Trim
    the bell peppers' bottoms to make
    sturdy bases, cut off the tops, and
    take out the seeds. Put the peppers
    in a baking dish after giving their
    exteriors a quick olive oil
    brushing.

    Heat up the veggies: Olive oil should be
3.
    heated to a medium temperature in a big

skillet. Sauté the chopped garlic and onions until they become tender.

4.   Chopped mushrooms should be added and cooked until they release moisture and turn golden brown.

5.   Cook the spinach until it wilts by stirring in the chopped spinach.

6. TossinguinoaorRiceandseason.

7.   Addsalt,pepper,anddriedthymetot he mixture to season. Stir thoroughly after adding the cooked rice or quinoa.

8. Includetheblackbeans:Stirtherinsed and drained black beans into the pan. Mix everything up thoroughly by stirring.

9. HowtoStuffBellPeppers:Gentlypress down on the prepped bell peppers as you spoon in the mushroom, spinach, and quinoa/rice combination.

10.   Addtomatosauceontop:Drizzle the stuffed peppers with tomato sauce,

making sure to coat them well.

11. Optional: Incorporate Vegan Cheese:
Top each stuffed pepper with a
sprinkling of vegan cheese if
using.

12. Bake: Once the oven is
preheated, bake the baking dish
covered with foil for 25

to 30 minutes, or until the peppers are soft.

13. Add a garnish and serve: Before serving, if preferred, sprinkle with fresh cilantro or parsley.

14. Enjoy: Serve the Mushroom and Spinach Stuffed Bell Peppers hot and enjoy your flavorful and hearty meal!

Feel free to customize the filling by adding your favorite herbs, spices, or additional vegetables. This dish is not only delicious but also a great way to incorporate a variety of nutritious ingredients.

## Vegan Buddha Bowl

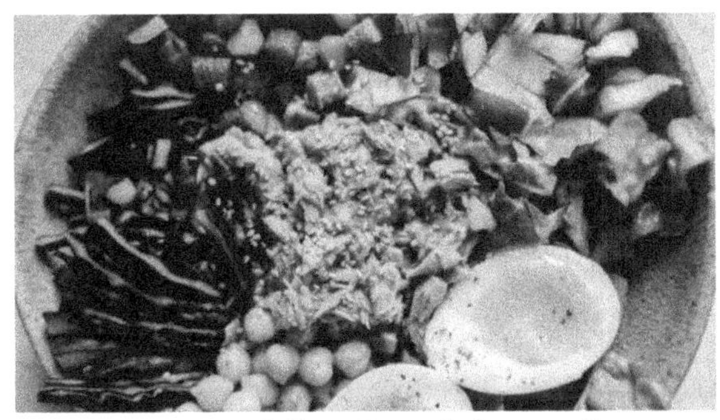

A Vegan Buddha Bowl is a vibrant

and nourishing dish that typically consists of a variety of plant-based ingredients arranged in a bowl. Here's a basic recipe to create a

delicious and visually appealing Vegan
Buddha Bowl:

Ingredients:

For the Base:

B
guinoaorbrownrice(cooke
d)                              B
Mixedgreensorspinach
For the Protein:

B
Chickpeas(roastedorsautée
d)                              B
Tofu(bakedorpan-fried)
B
Tempeh(marinatedandgrilled)
For the Vegetables:
B        Roastedsweetpotatoesorbutternut
squash
B
Steamedorroastedbroccoli
B Slicedavocado
O Shreddedcarrots

B

Cherrytomatoes,halved
B Cucumberslices

For the Dressing:

B
Tahinidressing,lemon-tahinidress
ing, or your favorite vegan
dressing Optional Toppings:

B
Sesameseeds
B Hempseeds
B Pumpkinseeds

B Freshherbs(cilantro,parsley)

Instructions:

1. Prepare the Base: Start by
   placing a portion of cooked
   quinoa or brown rice at the
   bottom of each bowl. Add a
   handful of mixed greens or
   spinach on tool

2. Add the Protein: Arrange your
   chosen protein source on one side
   of the bowl. This could be roasted

chickpeas, baked tofu, or grilled tempeh.

3. Include the Vegetables: Arrange a variety of colorful vegetables on the other side of the bowl. Some examples

of this include roasted sweet potatoes, steamed broccoli, sliced avocado, shredded carrots, cherry tomatoes, and cucumber slices.

4. Mixthedressingwiththedrizzle.

Drizzle the bowl with your preferred vegan dressing, such as lemon-tahini or

tahini. Another choice is a squeeze of fresh lemon juice.

5. Addanydesiredgarnishes:Addsome

sesame, hemp, or pumpkin seeds, or some fresh herbs like cilantro or parsley for added flavor and nutrients.

6. IntheNowandSavor:Youcannow

enjoy your vegan Buddha Bowl at last! Mix the ingredients together or savor each one separately.

Feel free to be creative and top your Buddha

Bowl with any plant-based ingredients you choose. Using a variety of colors, textures, and flavors is essential to creating an aesthetically appealing. In addition to being delicious, Buddha Bowls are an excellent way to get a variety of nutrients into one filling meal.

# Quesadillas with black beans and corn

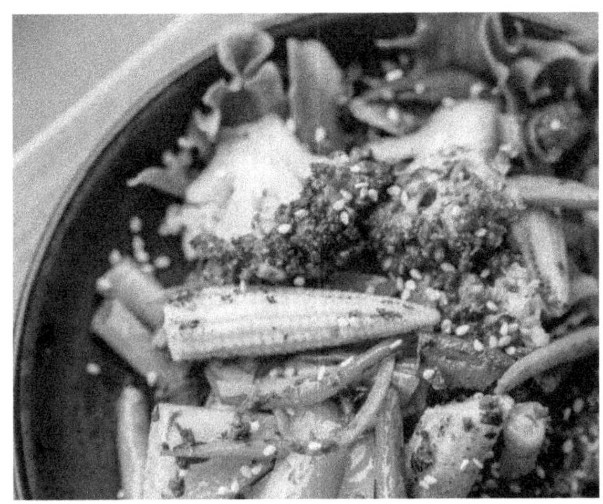

guesadillas with black beans and corn are tasty and filling, and they come together quickly. Here's a quick recipe that you will love:

Ingredients:

- One can (15 oz) of rinsed and drained black beans
- One cup of fresh, frozen, or canned corn kernels
- One chopped bell pepper

- Half a red onion, cut finely

Remove the seeds from one jalapeño and cut it finely (optional for heat).

One teaspoon of cumin powder

One tsp of chili powder

To taste, add salt and pepper.

One cup of vegan cheese (either a Mexican blend or cheddar) shredded

O   Four large corn or whole wheat tortillas

O   For cooking, use olive oil or cooking spray.

Guacamole, salsa, or vegan sour cream for serving (optional)

Instructions:

1.   Prepare the Filling: In a mixing bowl, combine black beans, corn, diced bell pepper, red onion, jalapeño (if using), ground cumin, chili powder, salt, and pepper. Mix well to combine.

2   Cook the Filling: Heat a non-stick skillet over medium heat. Add the bean and corn mixture to the skillet and cook for 5-7 minutes, stirring occasionally,

until the vegetables are softened and the mixture is heated through.

3. Assemble the guesadillas: Place a tortilla on a flat surface. Spoon a portion of the black bean and corn mixture onto one half of the tortilla. Sprinkle a generous amount of vegan cheese over the filling.

4. Fold the remaining tortilla half over the filling to form a half-moon shape.

5. Prepare the guesadillas: Cooking spray or a small bit of olive oil can be used to lightly coat the skillet. Cook for 2-3 minutes on each side, or until the tortilla is golden brown and the cheese has melted.

6. Repeat with the remaining tortillas.

Cut and Serve: Remove the quesadillas from the griddle and set them aside for a

7. minute to cool. Make slices out of each quesadilla.

8. Optional toppings: Serve with guacamole, salsa, vegan sour cream, or your favorite toppings.

9. Enjoy:Takepleasureinyours avoryand filling Black Bean and Corn guesadillas!

These quesadillas are a flexible and filling dish. Feel free to add additional vegetables or spices to your liking.

## Sweet Potato and Lentil Curry:

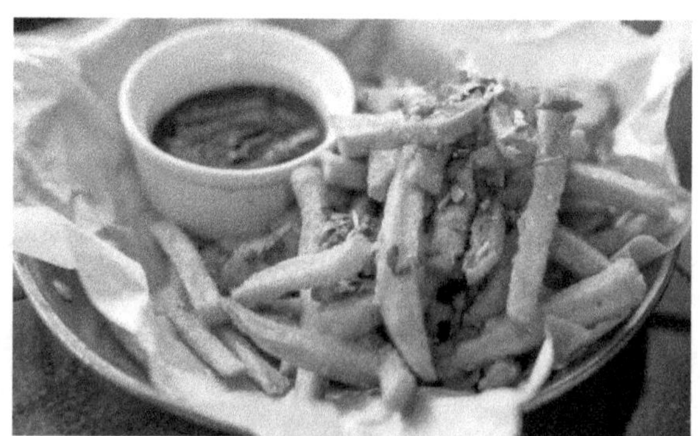

Sweet Potato and Lentil Curry is a tasty and nourishing recipe that is simple to prepare. Here's an easy recipe for you:

Ingredients:

1 cup rinsed and drained red or green lentils

☐    2 big sweet potatoes, peeled and chopped

1 onion, finely chopped 3 garlic cloves, minced

☐    1 tbsp grated fresh ginger

1 can (14 oz) chopped tomatoes

1 can (14 oz) coconut milk

2 tbsp curry powder 1tsp turmeric powder 1tsp cumin 1tsp paprika 1/2 teaspoon cinnamon

1/4teaspoon cayenne pepper (adjust to taste for heat)

☐ Season with salt and pepper to taste

n    Two tablespoons of coconut or vegetable oil for cooking

☐    Finely chopped fresh cilantro as a garnish

cooked naan or rice to be served

Guidelines:

1. Clean the Lentils: Lentils should be rinsed with cold water and left aside.

2. Aromatics in sauté: Cooking oil should be heated over medium heat in a big pot. Sauté the chopped onion until it turns transparent.

Add the grated ginger and minced garlic.

3. Sauté until aromatic, one or two more minutes.

4. Include Spices: To the pot, add the curry powder, ground cumin, ground turmeric, ground cinnamon, and cayenne pepper. To thoroughly mix the spices with the aromatics, stir well.

5. Prepare Sweet Potatoes and Lentils: Toss in the rinsed lentils, diced tomatoes, diced sweet potatoes, and coconut milk. Add pepper and salt for seasoning.

6. In order to blend all the components, stir.

7. After bringing the mixture to a boil, lower the heat to a simmer, cover it, and cook for 20 to 25 minutes, or until the sweet potatoes and lentils are soft.

8. Modifytheseasoning:Ifnecessary,
taste and adjust the seasoning by adding
extra salt or spices.

9. Serve:ServetheLentilandSweet

Potato Curry over Naan or over
boiled rice.

10. Accessory: Before serving,
add some freshly cut cilantro as a
garnish.

11. Enjoy:Savoryourtastyandnourishing
curry made with sweet potatoes and
lentils!

In addition to being tasty, this curry is also
high in fiber and protein. You can eat
this filling and cozy dinner by itself or
with your preferred side dishes.

## Vegan Sushi Rolls

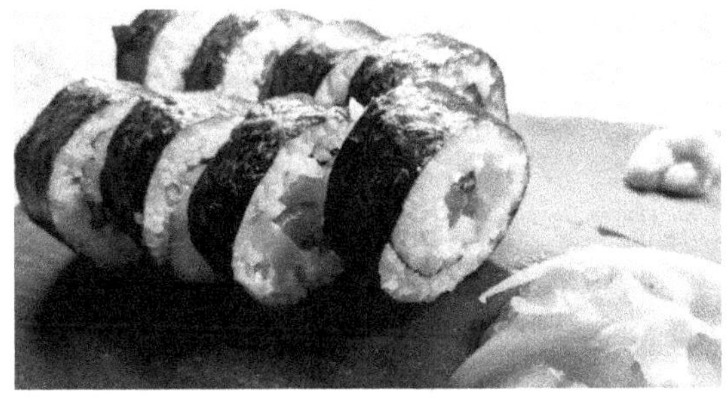

Enjoying this Japanese treat is made easy and tasty when you make vegan sushi rolls at home. Here's a basic recipe for vegan sushi rolls that include delicious ingredients like avocado and cucumber:

Ingredients:

Regarding the Sushi Rice:

B twocupsofsushirice

B
1/2cupricevinegarand21/2cups
water

B twotspsugar

B
Forthevegansushirolls,useone
teaspoon of salt.

B
Seaweed(nori)sheets

B sushirice

B Avocado,slicedcucumber,carrot,red

or yellow bell pepper, and black or white sesame seeds, finely chopped, as garnish

B Todip in Soy Sauce

B Wasabi and pickled ginger, for serving (optional)

Guidelines:

1    Assemble the sushi rice.

Till the water runs clear, rinse the sushi rice under cold water.

2
3.    In a rice cooker, combine rice with

water and cook as directed by the device.

4.    Mix the sugar, salt, and rice vinegar in a small pot. Stir the sugar and salt until they dissolve while heating over low heat. Allow it to cool.

5.    When cooked, pour the rice into a big basin. Using a wooden spatula, gradually fold the vinegar mixture into the rice. When the rice cools to room temperature, let it.

6    Assemble the fillings.

Cut the avocado into slices and finely chop the bell pepper, carrot, and

7  cucumber.



8. Put together the vegan sushi rolls: On a spotless surface, lay out a bamboo sushi rolling mat. Spoon a sheet of nori onto the mat, shiny side down.

9. Applyathinlayerofsushiric
etothe nori using wet fingers,
leaving about 1 inch at the top
border.

10. Layoutthebellpepper,cucumber,
avocado, and carrot slices in a
horizontal fashion on the bottom
third of the nori coated with rice.

11. Using the bamboo mat to help form it,
begin rolling the sushi away from
you. Use some water to seal the
edge.

12. Cutintopiecesandserve:Usinga
moistened sharp knife, cut the rolled
sushi into little pieces.

13. With the remaining materials,
repeat the procedure.

14. Add a garnish and serve: For a textural
contrast, top the sushi rolls with sesame
seeds.

15. Providesoysaucefordippingbesidethe
vegan sushi rolls. Add wasabi and
pickled ginger as an optional side
dish.

16. Enjoyyourself:Savoryourdelici
    ous and nourishing dinner of
    homemade
vegan sushi rolls!

You may use tofu, marinated
mushrooms, or other fresh vegetables
as fillings, so feel free

to get creative. You can personalize sushi when you make it at home.

## Chickpea and Spinach Coconut Stew

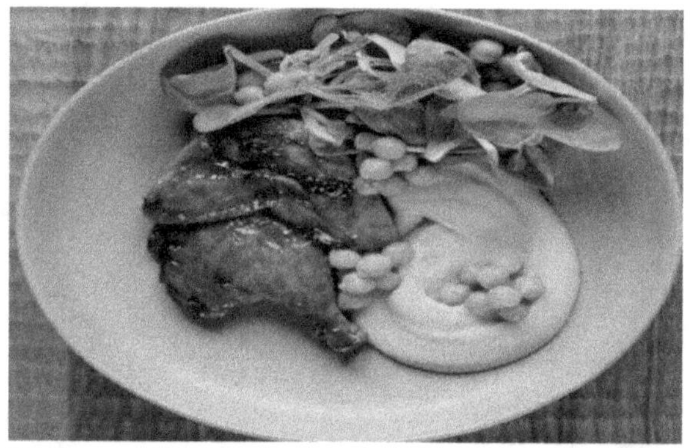

This recipe is cozy and savory, and it's really simple to make. I'll give you a quick recipe:

Ingredients list:

One fifteen-ounce can of rinsed and drained chickpeas

One finely sliced onion
minced three garlic cloves

one     tablespoon     grated
ginger

One can of diced tomatoes (14 oz.) One can of coconut milk (14 oz).

Four cups freshly chopped spinach One tsp of ground cumin

one tsp finely ground coriander One tsp finely ground turmeric

Half a teaspoon red pepper flakes (adjust for intensity, according to taste) To taste, add salt and pepper.

Two tablespoons of coconut or vegetable oil for cooking

Finely chopped fresh cilantro as a garnish

For serving, cooked rice or crusty bread

Guidelines:

1.   Aromatics in sauté: Cooking oil should be heated over medium heat in a big pot. Sauté the chopped onion until it turns transparent.

2. Add the grated ginger and minced garlic. Sauté until aromatic, one or two more minutes.

3. Include Spices: Toss in the red pepper flakes, ground cumin, ground coriander, and ground turmeric. To thoroughly mix the spices with the aromatics, stir well.

4. Prepare the chickpeas: Stir the chickpeas into the pot with the spices after adding them.

5. Add the coconut milk and tomatoes: Add the coconut milk and diced tomatoes. After giving it a good stir, simmer the mixture.
Reduce:To enable the flavors to merge, lower the heat to low, cover the pot, and simmer for 15 to 20 minutes.

7. Inc|udespinach:Inc|udefresh|y chopped spinach in the stew. As the spinach

wilts and becomes incorporated into the stew, stir it.

8. Modify the seasoning: Add pepper and salt to the stew to season it. If necessary, taste and adjust the seasoning.

9. Serve: Serve the Coconut Stew with Chickpeas and Spinach over crusty bread or over boiled rice.

10. Accessory: Before serving, add some freshly cut cilantro as a garnish.

11. Enjoy: Enjoy your delicious and nutritious Chickpea and Spinach Coconut Stew!

This stew is not only flavorful but also rich and satisfying. It's a perfect dish for a cozy and comforting meal.

## Mushroom and Walnut Tacos

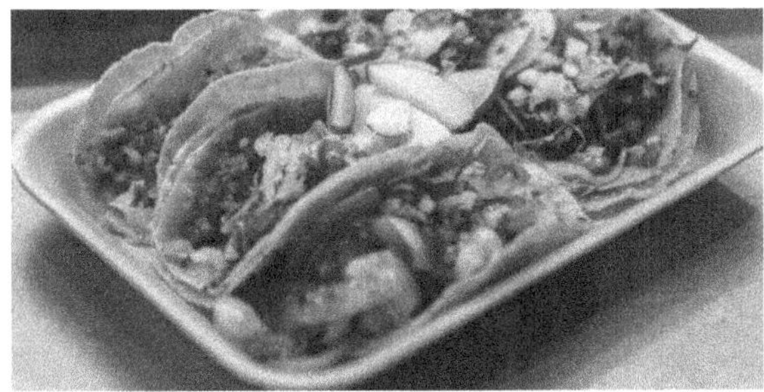

Mushroom and Walnut Tacos are a delicious and satisfying plant-based alternative to traditional meat tacos. Here's a simple recipe for you:

Ingredients:

For the Mushroom and Walnut Filling:

2 cups mushrooms, finely chopped 6cup walnuts, finely chopped

6onion, finely chopped 6cloves garlic, minced 6tablespoon olive oil 6teaspoon ground cumin 6teaspoon smoked paprika 6teaspoon chili powder @lt and pepper to taste @ice of 1 lime For the Tacos:

B Cornorflourtortill
as              B Avocadoslices
B Shreddedlettuceorcabbag
e B Dicedtomatoes
B Freshcilantro,choppe
d B slicesoflime.
B Hotsauce,vegansourcream,andsal
sa are optional.

Guidelines:

1. Get ready to make the walnut and mushroom filling.

2. Add the olive oil to a skillet and heat it to medium. Once added, sauté the onions until they become transparent.

3. Put the chopped mushrooms and minced garlic in there. In order for the mushrooms to shed their moisture and becoming soft, cook them for five to seven minutes.

4. Add smoked paprika, chopped walnuts, chili powder, ground cumin, salt, and pepper. Stir the mixture and let the flavors mingle for a further 5 to 7 minutes of cooking.

5. Drizzle the filling with lime juice, then mix it in. Take the heat off.

6. Put together the tacos: Tequila should

be warmed according the directions on the packaging.

7. Fill each tortilla with a spoonful of the mushroom and walnut mixture.

8. Top with avocado slices, shredded
   lettuce or cabbage, diced tomatoes, and
chopped cilantro.

9. Add Optional Toppings: Drizzle with
   salsa, hot sauce, or vegan sour
cream if desired.

10. Serve: Serve the Mushroom and
    Walnut Tacos with lime
    wedges on the side.

11. Enjoy: Enjoy your flavorful and
protein-packed Mushroom and Walnut
Tacos!

Feel free to customize your tacos with
additional toppings like vegan cheese,
pickled onions, or jalapeños. These
tacos are a delicious and hearty option
for a plant- based meal.

# Vegan Mediterranean Bowl

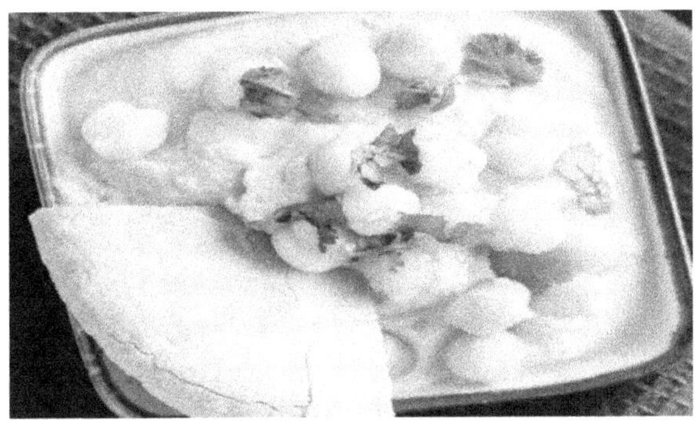

A Vegan Mediterranean Bowl is a colorful and nutritious dish that typically features a variety of fresh vegetables, grains, and flavorful sauces. Here's a simple recipe for you to create a delicious Vegan Mediterranean Bowl:

Ingredients list:

Concerning the Base:
B
1cupofbulgurwheatorcookedquinoa
B Twocupsofmixedgreensforsalad
(kale, spinach, arugula, etc.)
Concerning the Protein:

B
Onefifteen-ouncecanofrinsedand
drained chickpeas

# B Asinglespoonfulofoliveoil

One tsp of ground cumin

A single tsp of smoky paprika Add salt and pepper to taste. Concerning the Vegetables:

B Cherrytomatoes,cucumberscutinhalf, red onions cut thinly, pitted and sliced Kalamata olives

Concerning the Extras:

B HummusTzatzikisauce(vegan, or traditional, if desired)

B freshslicesoflemon

Optional garnishes:

B Crumbledveganfetacheese,choppe d fresh parsley

Guidelines:

1. Set Up the Foundation: Follow the cooking directions

on the package for bulgur wheat
or quinoa. Use a fork to fluff,
then set aside.

2.  In serving dishes, arrange mixed salad greens as the basis.

3   Spice up the chickpeas:

    Set oven temperature to 400°F, or 200°C.

4

5.  Combine chickpeas, smoked paprika, ground cumin, olive oil, and salt & pepper in a bowl. Place them on a baking sheet and roast for 20 to 25 minutes, or until they start to get golden and crisp.

6.  Put the BowlTogether:Toss in some cooked bulgur or quinoa and arrange it on top of each bowl's salad greens.

7.  Top with cherry tomatoes, cucumber slices, red onion slices, roasted chickpeas, and Kalamata olives.

8.  Include Extras: Transfer the vegan tzatziki sauce and hummus onto the bowls.

9. Decorative Add-ons: If preferred, top with crumbled vegan feta cheese and fresh parsley.

10.    Serve: Present the Vegan Mediterranean Bowls alongside freshly cut lemon wedges.

11.    Enjoy: Savor the flavors and colors of your vegan Mediterranean bowl!

Feel free to customize the bowl with your favorite Mediterranean ingredients, such as artichoke hearts, roasted red peppers, or marinated tofu. This versatile dish allows you to get creative and enjoy a variety of flavors and textures.

# CHAPTER SIX

## Snack Attack

### Guacamole and Veggie Sticks

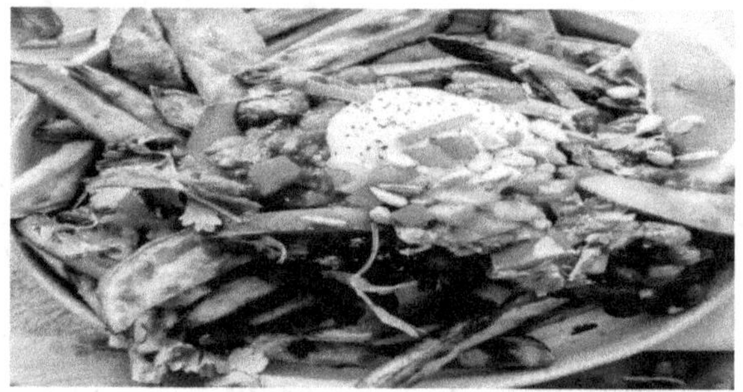

For a simple guacamole and veggie sticks: Guacamole:
Ingredients:

2 ripe avocados
1 lime §uiced)
1/4 cup red onion (finely chopped) 1 small tomato (diced)
1 clove garlic (minced)
Salt and pepper to taste
Fresh cilantro (chopped, optional)

Instructions:

1.     Scooptheavocadosintoa bowland mash them with a fork.
2. Addlimejuice,choppedredonion, diced tomato, minced garlic, salt, and pepper.
3. Mixuntilwellcombined.
4. Addchoppedcilantroifdesired.
5. Adjustsaltandpeppertotaste.

Veggie Sticks.

Additives:

Veg          sticks
Cucumber  stick
Bell         pepper
halves

Guide:

1. Peel and thinly slice the bell pepper, cucumber, and carrots into sticks or strips.
2  Place the vegetable sticks in a platter. As a tasty and nutritious snack, serve

3    the guacamole with the vegetable
     sticks. Take pleasure in!

# Whole grain crackers with Hummus

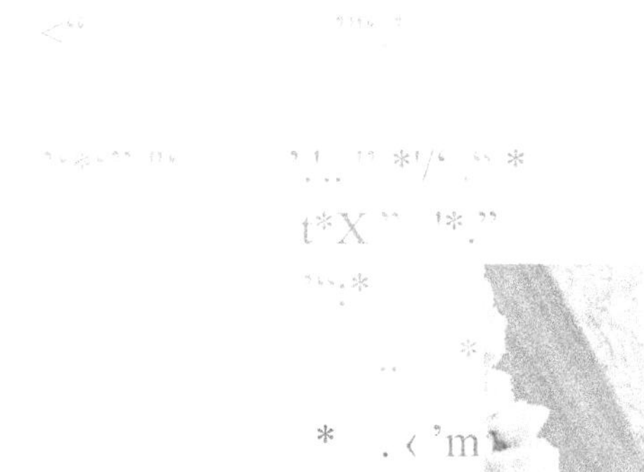

A tasty and healthful snack option is to make hummus with whole grain crackers.

Here's a basic recipe for homemade hummus to go with whole grain crackers:

Additives:

For the Hummus population:

B
Onefifteen-ouncecanofrinsedand drained chickpeas
B
1/4cupoffreshlysqueezedlemonjui ce, or roughly one large lemon
B
1/4cupofthoroughlymixedtah ini
B

Onelittlecloveofchoppedgarli
c

B

Twotablespoonsofextravirginoli
ve oil, plus additional for
serving

B 1/2tspgroundcumin

B Seasonwithsalttotaste

B  acoupleoftablespoonstothreeofwater

B Dashofpaprika,forserving(optional)

For Whole Grain Crackers:

B
1cupwholewheatflou
r B 1/4cuprolledoats
D1/4cupsesameseeds
D1/4cupfaxseeds
D1/4upunfowerseed
D1/4cuppumpkinseed
s D1/4cupo4veoi|
B 1/2cupwater
B 1/2teaspoonsalt
B Additionalseedsfortopping(optional)

Instructions:

1. Make Hummus:

a.      In a food processor, combine the chickpeas, lemon juice, tahini, minced garlic, olive oil, cumin, and a pinch of salt.

b.      Process the mixture until smooth, scraping down the sides of the bowl as needed.

c.      With the food processor running, add water, one tablespoon at a time, until the hummus reaches your desired consistency.

d.     Taste and adjust the seasoning by adding more salt or lemon juice if needed.

e. Pour the hummus onto a platter, top with a little olive oil and, if preferred, paprika.

2. Prepare Natural Grain Crackers:

a. Set the oven temperature to 175°C, or 350°F.

b. Put the rolled oats, sesame seeds, flaxseeds, sunflower seeds, and pumpkin seeds in a big mixing basin.

c. Combine the dry ingredients with salt, water, and olive oil. Stir to form a dough. A little additional water can be used if the dough seems too dry.

d. Using a floured surface, roll out the dough to the desired thickness.

e. Shape the dough into cracker shapes using a knife or cookie cutter.

f. Place the crackers on a baking sheet lined with parchment paper. If you like, sprinkle additional seeds on top.

g.      Bake in the preheated oven for about 12- 15 minutes or until the edges are golden brown.

h.      Allow the crackers to cool completely before serving.

3. Serve:

a.      Arrange the whole grain crackers on a serving platter alongside the bowl of hummus.

b.      Enjoy the hummus with the whole grain crackers as a tasty and nutritious snack.

Feel free to customize the recipe to suit your taste preferences, and enjoy this wholesome and satisfying snack!

## Fruit Smoothie Bowl

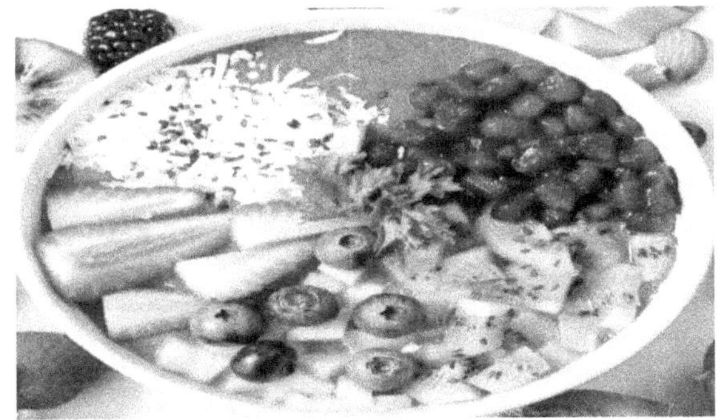

Creating a delicious fruit smoothie bowl is not only a treat for your taste buds but also a visually appealing and nutritious meal.

Here's a basic recipe to help you create a cool fruit smoothie bowl:

Ingredients:

Regarding the Smoothie:

B 0nefrozenbanana,cut
B
Onecupoffrozenberrymixture
(raspberries, blueberries, and
strawberries)
B halfacupofGreekyogurt,plain
B
1/4cupalmondmilk(oranyotherty
pe of milk)
B Onetablespoonofhoneyormaple
syrup (optional, based on desired
level of sweetness)
B
0neteaspoonofchiaseeds(optional;
adds extra nutrients and texture)

Regarding toppings:

B
slicedfreshfruit,suchasbananas,ki
wis, and berries
B granola
B
choppednuts,suchaswalnutsand

almonds
B
coconutshreds
B Chiaseeds
B Maplesyruporhoneytodrizzle

Guidelines:

1. Get the smoothie ready:

a.	Place the frozen banana slices, Greek yogurt, almond milk, frozen mixed berries, and honey/maple syrup in a blender.

b.	Blend the ingredients until smooth and creamy. If needed, add more almond milk in small amounts to achieve your desired consistency.

c.	Optionally, stir in chia seeds for added texture and nutritional benefits.

## 2. Assemble the Smoothie Bowl:

a. Pour the smoothie into a bowl.
b.	Smooth the surface with a spoon or spatula to create an even base.

## 3. Add Toppings:

a.	Arrange a variety of sliced fresh fruits, granola, chopped nuts, shredded coconut, and chia seeds on top of the smoothie base.

b.	Be creative with the arrangement to make it visually appealing.

4. Drizzle with Sweetener:

a.     If desired, drizzle honey or maple syrup over the top for a touch of sweetness.

5. Serveand Enjoy:

a.      Take a spoon and start eating! Combine the toppings with the smoothie base to create a delicious blend of textures and flavors.

You are welcome to add your preferred fruits, nuts, seeds, and other toppings to your smoothie bowl. In addition to being delicious, smoothie bowls are an excellent way to include a variety of nutrients into your diet. Savor this colorful and nutrient- dense breakfast or snack!

## Roasted Chickpeas

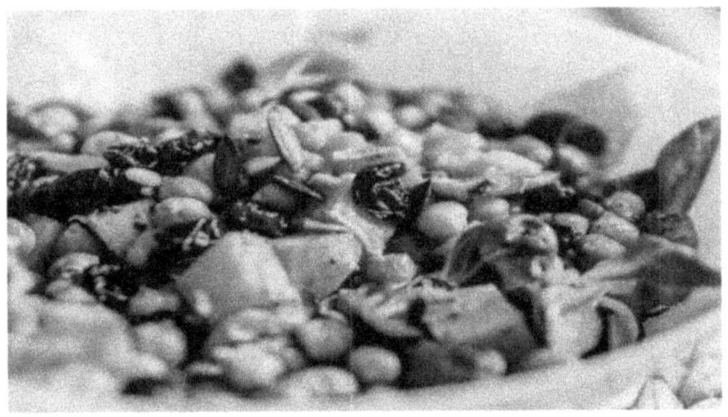

Chickpeas that have been roasted are a tasty and crunchy snack or a versatile addition to salads, bowls, and other

dishes. The following is a basic recipe
for roasted chickpeas:

Ingredients:

One can (15 oz) rinsed and drained chickpeas (garbanzo beans)
One or two teaspoons of olive oil
One teaspoon of cumin powder
One tsp of smoky paprika
half a teaspoon of powdered garlic Half a teaspoon of powdered onion Half a teaspoon of chili powder (add more or less to taste)
To taste, add salt and pepper.

Guidelines:

1. Warm up the oven: Set oven temperature to 400°F, or 200°C.

2. Dehydrated Chickpeas: Using a fresh kitchen towel or paper towels, pat dry the washed and drained chickpeas. For crispier results, excess moisture must be removed.

3 Toss the chickpeas:The dry chickpeas should be combined with

olive oil, chili powder, smoked paprika, ground cumin, garlic powder, onion powder, and salt and pepper in a dish. Make sure the seasoning coats the chickpeas evenly.

4. Disperse onto a baking sheet: Arrange the seasoned chickpeas on a baking pan in a single layer. To ensure uniform roasting, make sure they are not packed too tightly.

5. Baked Roast: The chickpeas should be roasted for 20 to 30 minutes, or until they are crispy and golden brown. To ensure consistent cooking, shake the baking sheet or stir the chickpeas halfway through the roasting process.

6. When the chickpeas are roasted, take them out of the oven and allow them to cool on the baking sheet. When they cool, they will keep getting crispier.

7. Serve: Roasted chickpeas can be added as a crispy garnish to salads, soups, or bowls, or served as a snack.

8. Store: Any leftover roasted chickpeas should be kept at room temperature in
an airtight container. For greatest crispiness, they are best consumed within a day or two of preparation.

9. Enjoy yourself: Savor your healthy, high-protein snack or add crispy texture to a variety of foods with your handmade roasted chickpeas!

You are welcome to experiment with different seasonings to suit your own tastes. Not only are roasted chickpeas a delicious but healthful substitute for store-bought snacks.

# Fruit Salad with Mint

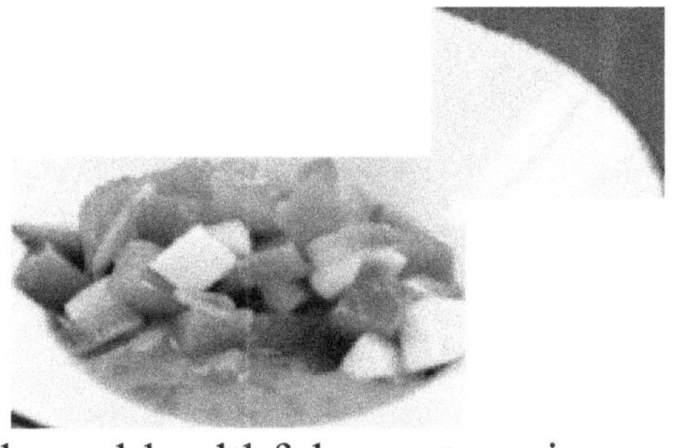

A lovely and healthful way to enjoy a variety of fruits is with a refreshing fruit salad with mint. I'll give you a quick recipe:

Ingredients list:
Concerning the Fruit Salad:

B    Halfacupandahulloffresh strawberries

B onecupofrawblueberries
B
Onecupoffreshlycutpineapple
B Onecupoffreshlycutgrapes

a pair of peeled and sliced kiwi fruits One orange, separated and peeled

Concerning the Mint Syrup:

B 1/4cupfreshlychopped,finelychopped mint leaves D1/4cupmap|esyruporhoney B twoteaspoonsoflemonorlimejuice, fresh

Guidelines:

1. Get the Fruit Ready: As needed, wash and prepare each fruit. Chop them up into small pieces and transfer them to a big mixing basin.

2. How to Make Mint Syrup: Chopped mint leaves, honey, maple syrup, and fresh lime or lemon juice should all be combined in a small basin. Mix thoroughly by stirring.

3. To make mixing simpler, you might want to slightly warm the honey if using it.

4 Toss the salad of fruit.

Transfer the mint syrup to the mixing bowl with the prepared fruits.

5

6.    Tossthefruitsgentlysothe
mintsyrup coats them evenly.

7.  Chill:Beforeserving,thefruitsal
    ad should be chilled for at
    least half an hour. Chilling
    allows the flavors to
meld and enhances the freshness.

8.    Serve:3ustbeforeserving,gi
    vethefruit salad a gentle stir. You
    can also garnish
it with additional fresh mint leaves if
desired.

9.    Enjoy:Enjoyyourrefreshi
ngFruit Salad with Mint as a
light and healthy snack or
dessert.

Feel free to customize the fruit
selection based on what's in season or
your personal preferences. This fruit
salad is not only delicious but also a
visually appealing and nutritious treat.

# Trail Mix

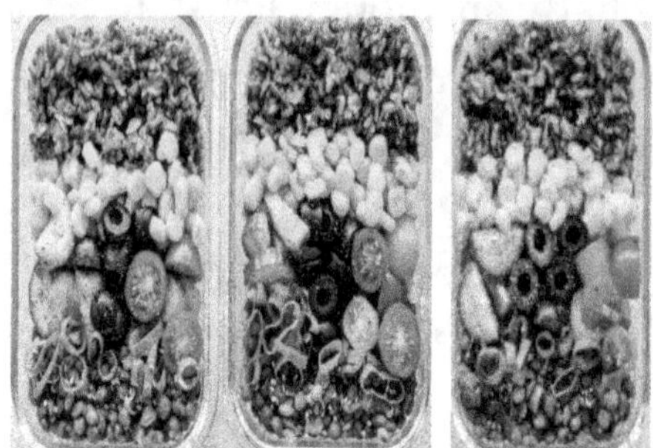

Trail mix is a versatile and energy-boosting snack that combines a variety of nuts, seeds, dried fruits, and sometimes chocolate or other sweet elements. Here's a basic recipe for a homemade trail mix, but feel free to customize it according to your preferences.

Ingredients list:

1-cup raw or roasted almonds 1-cup raw or roasted walnuts

1-cup raw or roasted cashews

One cup of seeds from pumpkins

Dried cranberries, one cup One cup golden or raisins

One cup of dark chocolate chunks or chips, if desired

One cup of unsweetened shredded coconut

One tsp sea salt (optional, for a savory- sweet combination)

Guidelines

1. Pick and Prepare the Ingredients: Select the nuts and seeds that you prefer. Should you choose to use raw nuts, you can toast them for a few minutes over medium heat in a dry skillet until they get aromatic. Let them come to room temperature.

2. Mix the Ingredients: Combine the almonds, cashews, walnuts, raisins, pumpkin seeds, dried cranberries, dark chocolate chips, and shredded coconut in a big

bowl.

3. Add Salt (Optional): If you prefer a sweet-savory mix, you can add a teaspoon of sea salt. Toss the mixture to evenly distribute the salt.

4. MixWell:Mixalltheingredientswell
to ensure an even distribution of flavors.

5.      Store:Transferthetrailmixto
an airtight container or divide it
into smaller snack-sized bags for
on-the-go convenience.

6.      Enjoy:Enjoyyourhomema
detrailmix   as   a   quick   and
satisfying snack. It's
perfect for hiking, road trips, or a
boost of energy between meals.
Customization Tips:

7. NutsandSeeds:Feelfreetomixand
match your favorite nuts and seeds,
such   as   pistachios,   pecans,
sunflower
seeds, or chia seeds.

8.      DriedFruits:Swapoutthedri
ed cranberries and raisins for
alternatives
like dried apricots, mango, or pineapple.

9.      SweetElements:Custo
mizethe sweetness by adding
or   omitting   chocolate   or

choosing a variety of chocolate (dark, milk, white).

10. Spices:Experimentwithspi ceslike cinnamon or nutmeg for added flavor.

Trail mix is highly customizable, so feel free to get creative and tailor it to your taste preferences.

## Nut Butter and Banana Slices:

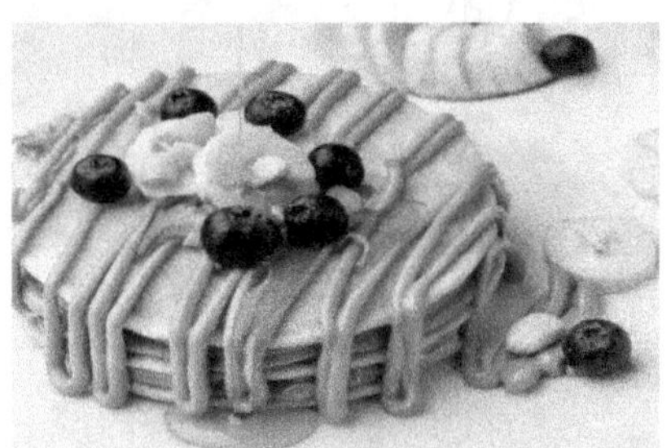

Nut butter and banana slices make for a delicious and nutritious snack that's quick and easy to prepare. Here's a simple recipe for this tasty treat:

Ingredients:

- ☐ 1 ripe banana
- ☐ 2 tablespoons nut butter (peanut butter, almond butter, or your favorite)
- ☐ Optional toppings: Chia seeds, hemp seeds, sliced strawberries, drizzle of honey

or maple syrup

Guidelines:

1. Cutthebananaintoslices:Afte
rpeeling, cut the ripe banana into
rounds. Slices can be cut to the
desired thickness.

2. DistributeNutButter:Placeasmall
   coating of your preferred nut butter
over each slice of banana. For even
spreading, use the back of a spoon
or a butter knife.

3. Add-ontoppings:Forextratexture
   and nutritional value, you can
   also top the
nut butter with hemp or chia seeds.

4. PutTogether:Placethebanan
aslicesin a serving dish or plate.

5. Drizzle0ptional:Youcansprinklea
   little honey or maple syrup over the
banana slices for an added touch of
sweetness.

6. Enjoy:Savoryourbananasli
ceswith nut butter as a healthy
snack!

This snack is not only delicious but also provides a good balance of natural sugars from the banana, healthy fats from the nut butter, and additional nutrients from optional toppings. It's a great choice for a quick energy boost or a satisfying treat.

## Rice Cake with Avocado:

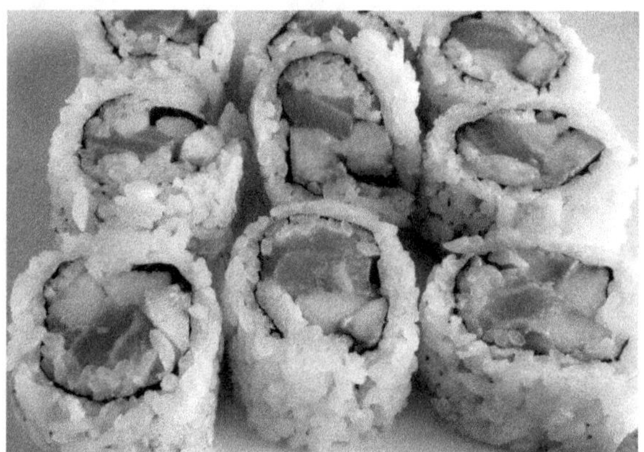

A Rice Cake with Avocado is a simple and nutritious snack that's easy to make. Here's a basic recipe for you:

Ingredients:

1 rice cake (plain or lightly salted) 1/2 ripe avocado
Salt and pepper, to taste

Optional toppings: Red pepper flakes, sesame seeds, drizzle of olive oil, lime or lemon juice

Instructions:

1. Prepare the Avocado: Cut the ripe avocado in half, remove the pit, and scoop the flesh into a bowl.

2. Blend the Avocado: Mash the avocado with a fork until it has the consistency you want. It can be smoothed out or left quite chunky.

3. Add some spice to the avocado: To taste, add salt and pepper to the mashed avocado. Stir thoroughly.

4. Apply to Rice Cake: Evenly cover the rice cake with the seasoned

mashed
avocado.

5. Extra Toppings at Option: You
may personalize your rice cake
by adding

extra toppings like sesame seeds, red pepper flakes, olive oil drizzling, or a squeeze of lemon or lime.

6.      Serve:Servethericecakewit havocado right away after plating it.

7.      Enjoyyourself:Savoryourr icecake with avocado for a light and nutritious snack!

This snack is not only delicious but also provides a good source of healthy fats from the avocado and complex carbohydrates from the rice cake. It's a versatile recipe, and you can get creative with additional toppings or variations based on your preferences.

# Vegetable Spring Rolls

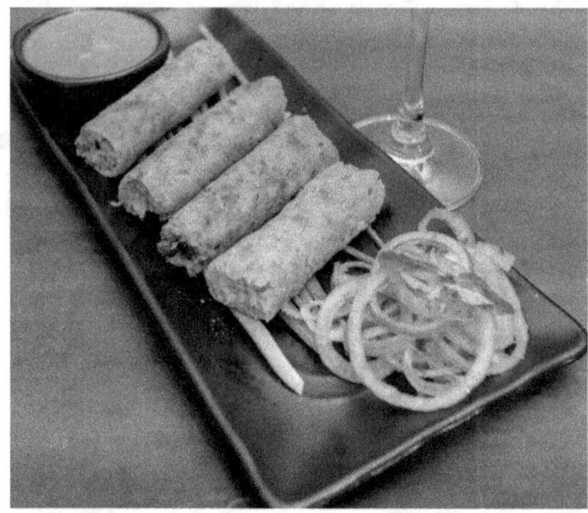

Vegetable spring rolls are a delicious and light appetizer or snack. Here's a simple recipe to make homemade vegetable spring rolls:

Ingredients:

For the Spring Rolls:

B  Ricepaperwrappers(springroll wrappers)
B
1cupricevermicellinoodles,cook ed and cooled

6cup    shredded    lettuce
6cup    julienned    carrots
6cup cucumber, julienned
6cup  red  bell  pepper,  julienned
Desh mint leaves
Desh cilantro leaves

For the Dipping Sauce:

B
1/4cupsoysauceortamari(fo
ra gluten-free option)
B
2tablespoonshoisinsauc
e                                    B
1tablespoonricevinegar
B
1teaspoonsesameoil
B  1teaspoonsugar
B  Redpepperflakes(optional,forheat)
B  Choppedpeanutsforgarnish(optional)

Instructions:

1.  Prepare the Ingredients: Cook the
    rice vermicelli noodles according
    to  the  package  instructions,  then
    cool and set aside.

2.   3ulienne the carrots, cucumber, and red bell pepper into thin strips.

3.   Prepare a shallow bowl of warm water for softening the rice paper wrappers.

4.   Soften Rice Paper Wrappers: Dip one rice paper wrapper into the warm water

for about 5-10 seconds until it becomes pliable but not too soft. Place it on a
clean, flat surface.

5. AssembletheSpringRolls:Onthe lower third of the rice paper, place a small handful of rice vermicelli noodles,
followed by lettuce, carrots, cucumber, red bell pepper, mint leaves, and cilantro.

6. Foldthesidesofthericepape rinand tightly roll up from the bottom, sealing
the edges. Repeat with the remaining ingredients.

7. MaketheDippingSauce:Inasmall bowl, whisk together soy sauce (or tamari), hoisin sauce, rice vinegar,
sesame oil, sugar, and red pepper flakes if using.

8. Serve:Arrangethevegetabl espring rolls on a serving plate and serve with the dipping sauce.

9.     0ptionalGarnish:Garnish with chopped peanuts for extra crunch.

10.   Enjoy: Enjoy your homemade Vegetable Spring Rolls as a tasty and refreshing appetizer!

These spring rolls are not only delicious but also customizable. You can add or substitute ingredients like tofu, avocado, or other fresh herbs to suit your taste. They are perfect for a light and healthy snack or as part of a meal.

## Vegan Energy Balls:

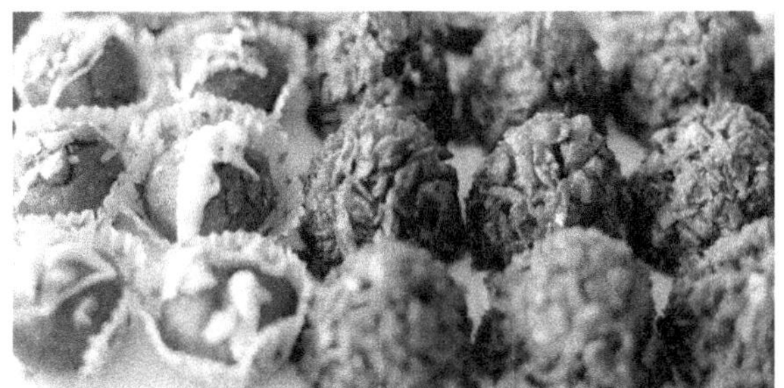

Vegan energy balls are a delicious and nutritious snack that is easy to make and perfect for a quick energy boost. Here's a simple recipe for homemade vegan energy balls:

Ingredients:

- 1 cup rolled oats
- 1/2 cup nut butter (almond

butter, peanut butter, or your favorite)

☐ 1/3 cup maple syrup or agave nectar ☐ 1/2 cup ground flaxseed

☐ 1/2 cup shredded coconut (unsweetened)

1 teaspoon vanilla
extract A pinch of salt
Optional add-ins: Chia seeds, hemp
seeds, chopped nuts, dried fruit,
cocoa powder

Instructions:

1. Combine Ingredients: In a large
   mixing bowl, combine rolled oats,
   nut butter, maple syrup or agave
   nectar, ground flaxseed, shredded
   coconut, vanilla extract, and a pinch
   of salt.

2. Mix Thoroughly: Mix the
   ingredients thoroughly until well
   combined. The mixture should be
   sticky enough to hold together.

3. Add Optional Add-Ins: If desired,
   add optional add-ins such as chia
   seeds, hemp seeds, chopped nuts,
   dried fruit,
   or cocoa powder for extra flavor
   and texture.

4. Chill the Mixture: Place the

mixture in the refrigerator for about 30 minutes. Chilling will make it easier to form the energy balls.

5. Form Energy Balls: Once the mixture has chilled, take small portions and roll

them between your hands to form bite- sized balls.

6. Store: Place the energy balls on a plate or tray and store them in the refrigerator for longer shelf life.

7.     Enjoy: Enjoy your Vegan E nergyBalls as a quick and nutritious snack!

These energy balls are not only tasty but also packed with fiber, healthy fats, and natural sugars to provide a sustained energy boost. Feel free to get creative with the ingredients and adjust the sweetness or texture to your liking.

## Oat and Nut Bars:

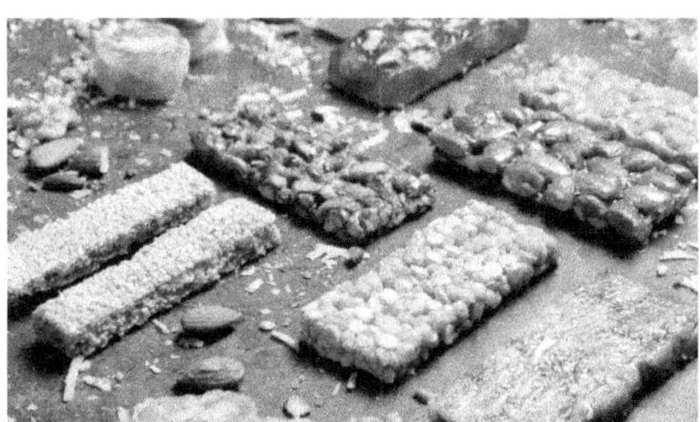

Oat and nut bars are a wholesome and satisfying snack that's easy to prepare. Here's a simple recipe for homemade oat and nut bars.

Ingredients list:

Two cups of traditional rolled oatsone cup chopped mixed nuts (almonds, walnuts, and cashews).

g   Half a cup of nut butter, either peanut butter or almond butter, is fine.
half a cup of maple syrup or honey

One-fourth cup melted coconut oil
one tsp vanilla essence
One-half teaspoon of optional cinnamon a small amount of salt

Guidelines:

1.  Warm Up the Oven: Set the oven temperature to 175°C/350°F. With an overhang on the sides for effortless removal, line a square or rectangular baking dish with parchment paper.

2.  Blend the dry ingredients together: Place the chopped mixed nuts and rolled oats in a large bowl.

3.  Assemble the moist ingredients: Melt the coconut oil in a different microwave- safe bowl or over the stove. Add the vanilla essence, nut butter,
honey (or maple syrup), and a small amount of salt.

4   Stir until thoroughly blended.

Mix the wet and dry ingredients together: After adding the wet

5   components to the dry ingredients, stir everything together until it is all coated.

6.  Put into the Baking Dish: Spoon the batter into the prepared baking dish. Using the back of a spoon or your hands, press it down evenly and firmly.

7.  Bake: The edges should get

golden brown after 15 to 20 minutes of baking in a preheated oven.

8. Aftercooling, cut: Let the bars in the baking dish cool fully. After the bars cool, pull the excess parchment paper to take them out of the dish. Transfer them to a cutting board, then cut into squares or bars.

9.   Store:Forextendedfreshness ,keepthe oat and nut bars chilled or store them in an airtight container at room temperature for a few days.

10.   Enjoy: Savor these healthy, on-the-go homemade Oat and Nut Bars!

You may personalize these bars by mixing in some chocolate chips, nuts, or dried fruits before baking. They're the ideal snack or rapid energy boost.

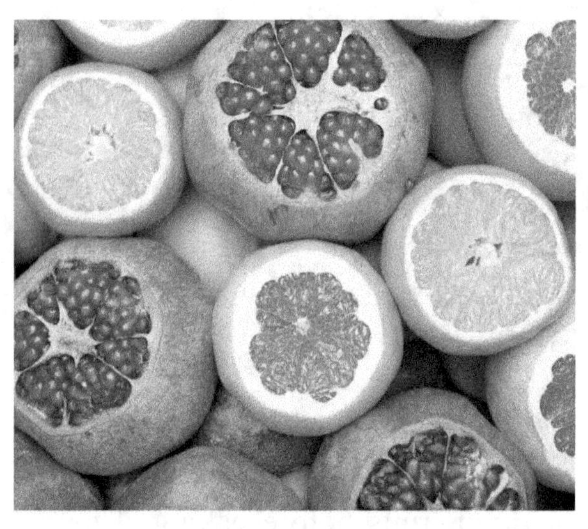

# CHAPTER SEVEN

## Sweet Treats/Desserts

### Vegan Chocolate Cake

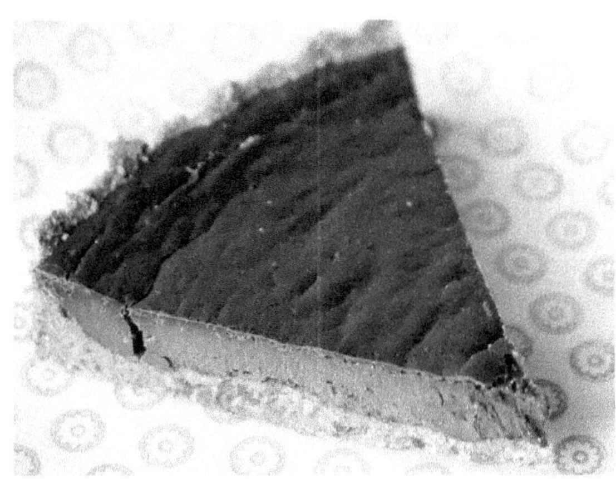

A delicious way to savor a traditional dessert without consuming any animal products is to make a vegan chocolate cake. This is a quick and delectable vegan chocolate cake recipe:

Additives:

Desiccated Components

B
Oneandahalfcupsofall-purposeflour
B 0necupofsugar,granulated
B
One-thirdcupofunsweetenedcocoa
powder
B
3ustonetspbakingsoda
B 1/2teaspoonsalt


Wet Ingredients:

B
0necupofplainalmondmilk(oran
y other plant-based milk)
B
Halfacupofmeltedcoconutoilor
vegetable oil
B Applecidervinegar,twotablespoons

B
ChocolateGanache(Optional):1tsp
vanilla extract

B

1/2cupchocolatechipswithoutdairy
B   1/4cupplant-basedmilk(coconutor otherwise).

## Guidelines:

1.      Turn on the oven: Set the oven temperature to 175°C/350°F. Coat a cake pan (8 or 9 inches) with butter and flour.

2.      Blend the dry ingredients: Add the flour, sugar, baking soda, cocoa powder, and salt to a large mixing bowl and whisk to combine.

3.      Mix Wet Ingredients Together: Mix the almond milk, vegetable oil, apple cider vinegar, and vanilla extract in a another bowl. Stir thoroughly.

4.      Mix the Dry and Wet Ingredients: Fill the dry ingredient bowl with the wet ingredients. Just blend by stirring. Don't overmix, please.

5. Grease: Using the prepared cake pan, pour the batter. Spread a spatula over the top. As soon as a toothpick inserted into the center comes out clean, bake for 25 to 30 minutes in a preheated oven.

5.      Awesome:When the cake is almost cool, take it out of the pan and place it on a wire rack to finish cooling.

6.    Construct       the       optional
chocolate  ganache:  Chocolate  chips
and coconut milk should be heated in
a small saucepan or microwave- safe
bowl until the chocolate is melted. Stir
until a smooth consistency is achieved.

7.    Cover the Cake: Apply the chocolate ganache on top of the cake after it has cooled fully.

8.    Arrange and Savor: Slice the cake and serve. This vegan chocolate cake is delicious on its own or with a scoop of dairy-free ice cream.

Feel free to get creative with the toppings or add-ins like chopped nuts, berries, or shredded coconut. Enjoy your cruelty-free and indulgent vegan chocolate cake!

# Coconut Milk Ice Cream

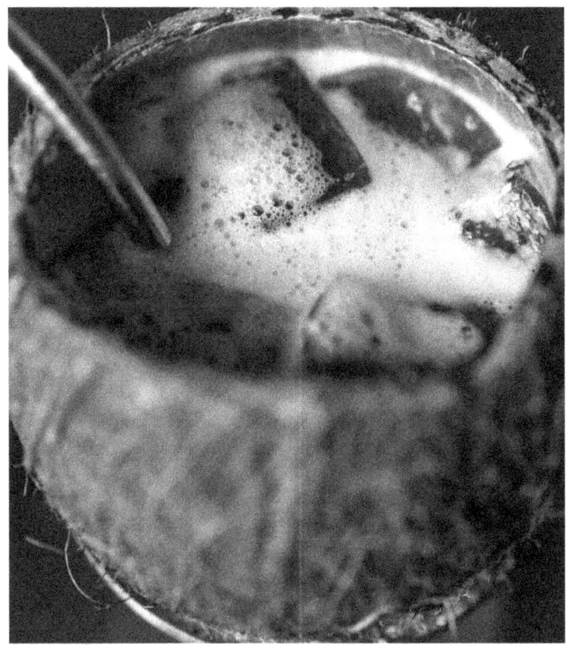

Making coconut milk ice cream is a wonderful way to enjoy a dairy-free, vegan treat. Here's a simple recipe for homemade coconut milk ice cream:

Ingredients:

☐   2 cans (27 ounces) full-fat coconut milk ☐   3/4 cup granulated sugar or sweetener

of choice (adjust to taste) ☐   1   teaspoon

vanilla extract □     Pinch
of salt

Optional: Flavorings or mix-ins (e.g., chocolate chips, crushed nuts, fruit)

Instructions:

1.     Chill the Coconut Milk: The coconut milk cans should be refrigerated for at least four hours or overnight. This aids in separating the liquid and cream.

2.     Set up the ice cream machine: Make sure the freezer bowl of your ice cream maker is frozen in accordance with the manufacturer's instructions if you have one.

3.     Take the Cream Out of the Liquid: Don't shake the cans of cold coconut milk when opening them. Remove the solid coconut cream from the top by spooning it out, discarding the liquid. About two cups of coconut cream should be consumed.

4.     Combine Components: Mix the coconut cream, sugar, vanilla essence, and a small amount of salt together in a mixing dish. Stir until sugar is completely dissolved.

5.     Movetheicecreamaround:Ifyou havean icecreammakerchrnthemixueunflM

achieves a soft-serve consistency by following the manufacturer's directions.

6.     Add any desired mix-ins:Stir in any optional mix-ins, like as fruit, chocolate
chips, or crushed nuts, in the last
five minutes of churning, if preferred.

7.     Moving to an Enclosure: Pour the churned ice cream into a container with a cover. You can freeze it for a few hours or overnight to get a harder texture.

8.     If you don't have an ice cream maker, use the hand-churning method: Pour the mixture into a freezer-safe container and store it
there if you don't have an ice cream machine. To get the appropriate consistency, use a fork to stir the liquid every thirty minutes to break up the ice crystals.

9.     Serve and Have Fun: When the ice cream has reached the consistency you choose, spoon it into bowls or cones

and serve.

This vegan coconut milk ice cream is very thick and creamy. Experiment with various flavor combinations to create a pleasant and dairy-free frozen treat!

# Cookies with almond butter

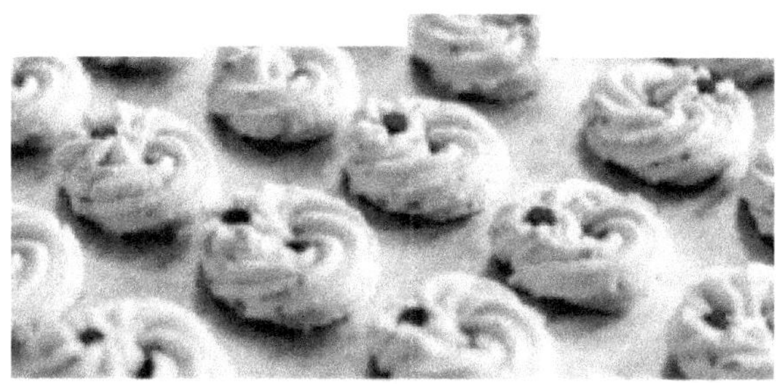

Almond butter cookies are a tasty and simple dessert. Here's an easy vegan almond butter cookie recipe:

Ingredients:

- ☐ 1 cup unsweetened almond butter
- ☐ 1/2 cup brown sugar or coconut sugar ☐ 1 flax egg (1 tbsp powdered flaxseed combined with 3 tbsp water, set aside for 5 minutes)
- ☐ a tsp vanilla extract
- ☐ a half teaspoon baking soda
- ☐ Optional: 1/4teaspoon salt 1/2 cup almonds or chocolate chips

Instructions:

1. Preheat the oven to 350°F: Start the oven at 175°C/350°F. Put parchment paper

on one baking sheet.

2.      Prepare your flax egg: The flax egg can be made by combining water and ground flaxseed in a small bowl. To make it thicker, leave it for roughly five minutes.

3.      Blend Wet Ingredients:Vanilla essence, flax egg, coconut sugar, and almond butter should all be combined in a mixing bowl. Mix thoroughly until well incorporated.

4.      Include the Dry Elements: The wet components should be combined with the baking soda and salt. Dough should come together after mixing.

5.      Add mix-ins if desired: Combine chocolate chips or chopped almonds with the cookie dough, if desired.

6.      Shape the Cookie Dough Balls: Shape the dough into balls by scooping out tablespoon-sized chunks.
On the baking sheet that has been prepared, arrange the balls, leaving some space between them.

6.    Flatten the cookies: Gently press a fork into each biscuit to make a crosshatch design.

7.    Prepare: Preheat the oven and bake for around 10 to 12 minutes, or until the sides get golden brown. Remember that baking

times could vary, so be sure to monitor the cookies to prevent overbaking.

8.      Cool: After a few minutes, let the cookies cool on the baking sheet before moving them to a wire rack to finish cooling.

9.      Enjoy: After the almond butter biscuits cool, savor them with your preferred non- dairy beverage or a glass of almond milk!

## Avocado Chocolate Mousse:

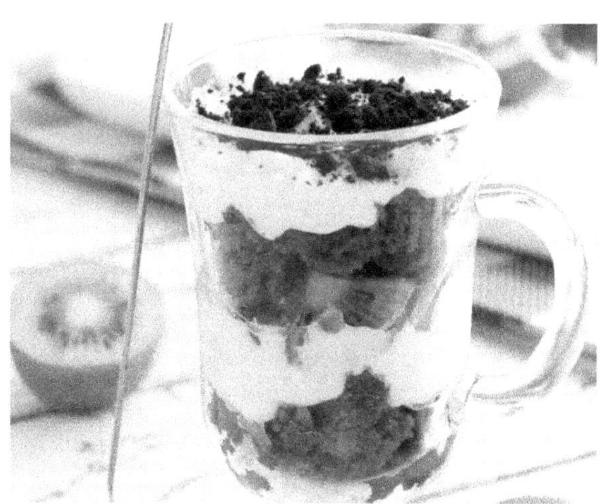

Here's a step-by-step guide on how to prepare Avocado Chocolate Mousse:

Ingredients:

0  two ripe avocados
0  1/4 cup of powdered cocoa

0   A quarter cup of honey or maple syrup,
    adjusted to taste

    Any non-dairy milk, including 1/4 cup almond
    milk

g   Measure out one teaspoon of vanilla
extract. g       A little teaspoon of salt
    Shaved chocolate, chopped nuts, or berries
    are optional garnishes.

Instructions:

1.  Get the avocados ready: Halve the
    avocados, remove the pit, and
    transfer the flesh to a food
    processor or blender.

2.  To the blender, add the
    ingredients: Add almond milk,
    vanilla extract, cocoa powder,
    honey, or maple syrup, and a small
    amount of salt to the blender.

3   Blend until smooth: Mix the
    ingredients until they are creamy
    and smooth. If necessary, scrape
    down the sides of the food
    processor or blender to make sure
    all the ingredients are thoroughly
    combined.

4.  Taste and Modify: Try the mousse and add extra honey or maple syrup to make it more sweet if necessary. If any
changes are made, blend once more.

5.     Chill:Toenablethechocolat emousse to cool and firm, transfer it to serving bowls or glasses and place them in the
refrigerator for at least half an hour. This improves the flavor even more.

6.     Add-ontoppings:Formorete xtureand flavor, you can top with optional ingredients like chopped nuts, berries,
or shaved chocolate before serving.

7. Serve:YourAvocadoChocolate
Mousse is ready to be served once it has been chilled and topped, if desired.

8. Enjoy:Savorthisdelectableand
healthful dessert choice, which is loaded with chocolate flavor and avocado's
creamy texture.

You are welcome to alter the recipe to suit your tastes. To suit your tastes, you can experiment with different toppings and change the mousse's sweetness and thickness.

# Vegan Cheesecake:

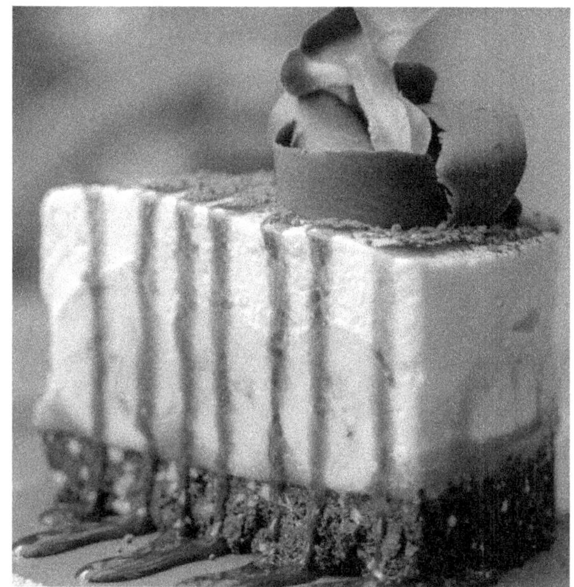

Vegan cheesecake is a delicious dairy-free alternative to traditional cheesecake. It often uses plant-based ingredients to create a creamy and flavorful dessert. Here's a simple recipe for a vegan cheesecake:

Ingredients:

For the Crust:

B 11/2cupsvegangrahamcracker crumbs (or other vegan cookie crumbs) B 1/4cupcoconutoil,melted

B
2tablespoonsmaplesyruporaga
ve nectar

Regarding the Filling:

B
Twocupsofuncookedcashewsthat
have been soaked in water for four
or
more hours
B 1/2cupmeltedcoconutoil
B Halfacupofcoconutmilk,fullfat
B
Halfacupofagavenectarormaple
syrup
B
one-fourthcuplemonjui
ce                        B
Onetspvanillaessence
B Asmallamountofsalt


Guidelines:

1.  Get the cashews ready: The raw
    cashews should be soaked in
    water for four hours or overnight.
    When not in use, drain and rinse

them.

2. Warm up the oven: Set the oven temperature to 350°F (175°C).

3. Prepare the Crust: Combine the melted coconut oil, maple syrup, and vegan graham cracker crumbs in a bowl and stir until completely blended.

4.      Tomakeauniformcrust,pr
essthe mixture firmly into the
bottom of a 9- inch springform
pan that has been
    greased or coated with parchment paper.

5.      ConcerningtheFilling:Two
cupsof raw cashews that have
been soaked in water for at least
four or all night

B Halfacupofmeltedcoconutoil
B
one-halfcupofcoconutmilk(full-f
at)                              B
1/2cupagavenectarormaplesyrup
B One-fourthcuplemonjuice
B
onetspvanillaessence
B
asmallamountofsalt
B guidelines:

6. Alignthecashews:Givetheraw
    cashews a minimum of four hours
or overnight soak in water. Before
usage, drain and rinse them.

7.      WarmUpthe0ven:Setth

eoven temperature to 175°C/350°F. 8.

9.      Tomakethecrust:Melttheco conutoil, add the maple syrup, and thoroughly
mix the vegan graham cracker crumbs in a bowl.

10.    Usinga9-inchspringformpan thathas been greased or coated with parchment

paper, press the mixture firmly into the bottom to achieve an equal crust.

11.    OptionalToppings:Garnishw ithfresh fruit, fruit compote, or a drizzle of chocolate sauce if desired.

12.    Enjoy: Enjoy your Vegan Cheesecake as a delicious and dairy-free dessert!

This vegan cheesecake is creamy, rich, and satisfying. It's a great option for those with dairy allergies or those following a plant- based diet.

## Oat Milk Panna Cotta:

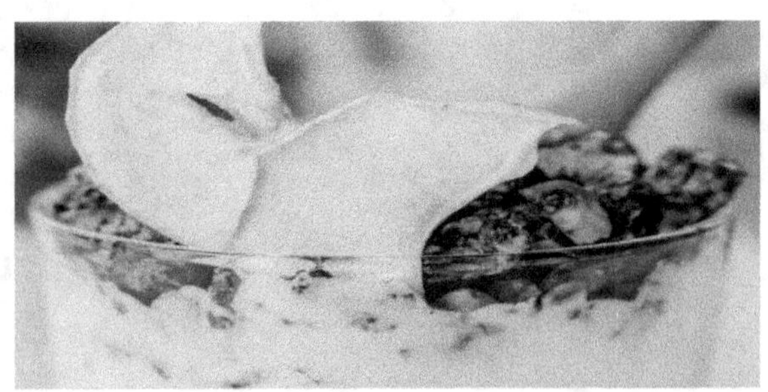

Oat milk panna cotta is a delightful dairy- free alternative to the traditional Italian dessert. It's smooth, creamy, and can be flavored in various ways. Here's a simple recipe for oat milk panna cotta:

Ingredients:

2 cups oat milk
1/4 cup maple syrup or agave nectar
1 teaspoon vanilla extract
2 teaspoons agar-agar powder (or 2 tablespoons agar-agar flakes)
Fresh berries or fruit compote for topping (optional)

Instructions:

1.  Get the Panna Cotta Base ready: Oat milk, vanilla extract, and maple syrup (or agave nectar) should all be combined in a pot. Over medium heat, whisk until thoroughly mixed.

2.  Incorporate Agar-Agar: To avoid

lumps, evenly sprinkle the agar-agar powder
(or pour the agar-agar flakes) over the oat milk mixture and whisk constantly.

3.  Warm and Low-Simmer: Over medium heat, bring the mixture to a moderate simmer. Once the agar-agar is completely dissolved, reduce the heat to medium and simmer, stirring constantly, for five to seven minutes.

4.  Calm A Little Bit: After taking the saucepan off of the burner, allow the mixture to cool for a short while.

5.  Pour into glasses or molds: Fill each mold or glass with the oat milk mixture.If using molds, lightly grease them with oil or cooking spray to facilitate easy removal.

6.  Chill: Place the molds or glasses in the refrigerator and let the panna cotta set for at least 4 hours or until fully chilled and firm.

7.  Serve: Once set, remove the panna

cotta from the molds or serve directly in
glasses.

8. Top with Berries (Optional): Top the oat milk panna cotta with fresh berries or a fruit compote just before serving.

9.    Enjoy:EnjoyyourOatMil
kPanna Cotta as a delicious and
dairy-free dessert!

Feel free to get creative with flavorings. You can infuse the oat milk with cinnamon, cardamom, or citrus zest for added depth. Oat milk panna cotta is a versatile dessert that accommodates various flavor profiles.

## Date and Nut Truffles:

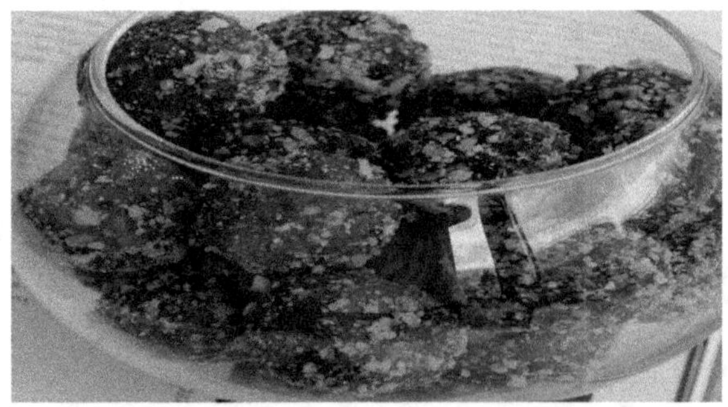

Date and nut truffles are a delicious and naturally sweetened treat that is simple to make. These energy-packed bites are perfect for a quick snack or a healthier dessert.

Here's a basic recipe:

Ingredients:

B 1cupdates,pitted

1 cup mixed nuts (such as almonds, walnuts, or cashews)
2 tablespoons cocoa powder (unsweetened)
1 teaspoon vanilla extract O A pinch of salt
Optional coatings: Shredded coconut, chopped nuts, cocoa powder

Instructions:

1. Prepare the Dates: If the dates are not soft, soak them in warm water for about 10 minutes to soften. Drain before using.

2. Mix Nuts: The mixed nuts should be combined in a food processor and pulsed until coarsely minced.

3. Add the cocoa and dates: Add the chopped nuts to a food processor along with the pitted dates, cocoa powder, vanilla extract, and a dash of salt.

4. Mix until well combined: Blend

the ingredients until a homogenous, sticky dough is formed. To guarantee even mixing, you might need to pause and scrape down the food processor's edges.

5.  Shape the truffle balls: To make bite-sized truffle balls, take tiny amounts of

the mixture and roll them between your palms.

6. TruffleCoat(Optional):For extrataste and texture, roll the truffles in your preferred coatings, such as chopped almonds, shredded coconut, or cocoa
powder.

7. Chill:Refrigeratethetruffles foratleast 30 minutes to harden up.

8. Serve:Servethedateandnuttruffles cold as a tasty and nutritious snack.

9. Store:Refrigerateanyremai ning truffles in an airtight container to keep them fresh.

10. Enjoy: As a pleasant and naturally sweet treat, enjoy your Date and Nut
Truffles!

You can change up the flavor of these truffles by adding ingredients like shredded coconut, chia seeds, or a pinch of cinnamon. They are an excellent alternative to store- bought sweets because they contain natural sweetness as well as healthy fats.

# Cups of Peanut Butter Chocolate:

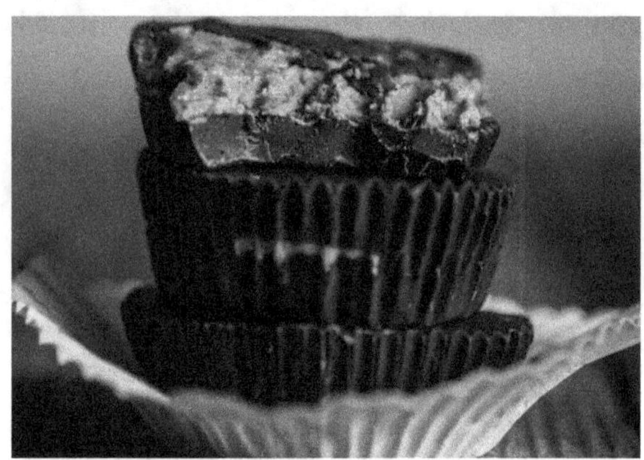

Peanut Butter Chocolate Cups are a traditional and decadent delicacy that is simple to create at home.

Here's a simple recipe for delicious Peanut Butter Chocolate Cups:

Ingredients:

- [ ] 1 cup chocolate chips (dark, semisweet, or a combination)
- [ ] 1/4 cup creamy peanut butter (or your favorite nut or seed butter)
- [ ] 2 tablespoons powdered sugar (optional, for sweetening the peanut butter)

Instructions:

1. Prepare Muffin Cups: Line a mini muffin tin with mini muffin cup liners.

2. Melt Chocolate: In a microwave-safe bowl or using a double boiler, melt the chocolate chips in 30-second intervals, stirring between each interval until fully melted and smooth.

3. Coat Muffin Cups: Spoon a small amount of melted chocolate into the bottom of each muffin cup, ensuring it covers the base.

4. Set Chocolate: Place the muffin tin in the refrigerator for a few minutes to allow the chocolate to set.

5. Prepare Peanut Butter Filling: In a separate bowl, mix the peanut butter with powdered sugar if you want to sweeten it.

6. Add Peanut Butter Layer: Take

a small amount of peanut butter mixture and roll it into a small ball. Flatten it slightly and place it on top of the set chocolate layer in each muffin cup.

7.   Cover with Chocolate: Spoon the remaining melted chocolate over the

peanut butter layer, covering it completely.

8.	Set in Refrigerator: Return the muffin tin to the refrigerator and let the Peanut Butter Chocolate Cups set completely. This usually takes about 30 minutes.

9. Serve:0nceset,removethePeanut Butter Chocolate Cups from the muffin tin and peel off the liners.

10.	Enjoy: As a delicious treat, serve your homemade Peanut Butter Chocolate Cups!

Add chopped nuts, sea salt, or even a coating of caramel between the chocolate and peanut butter to make these chocolate cups your own. Keep any leftover cups in the refrigerator to keep them fresh.

# Tiramisu vegano:

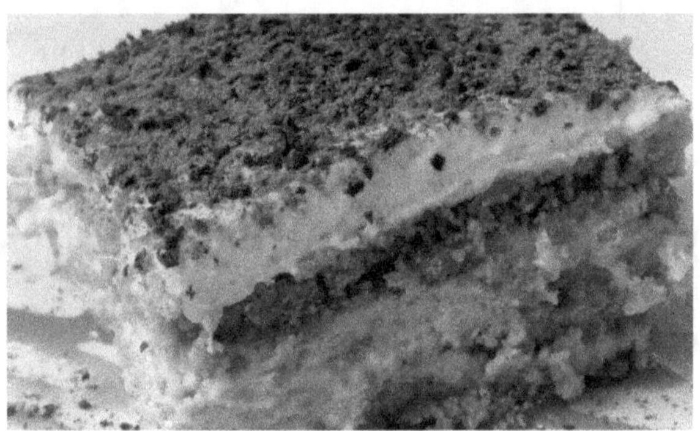

Vegan Tiramisu is a delectable dairy-free and egg-free variation of the traditional Italian dessert. Here's a quick and easy Vegan Tiramisu recipe:

Ingredients:

☐ Coffee Soaking Liquid

☐ 1 cup cooled, strong brewed coffee
☐ 2 tbsp coffee liqueur
☐ 2 tbsp maple or agave nectar ☐ Cashew Cream:

☐ 1 1/2 cup raw cashews, soaked in water for 4 hours or overnight

- ☐ 1/2 cup coconut cream (the thick portion of a full-fat coconut milk can)
- ☐ 1/2 cup agave nectar or maple syrup ☐ 1/4 cup coconut oil, melted

tsp vanilla extract
1-2 tablespoons lemon juice (according to taste)
grain of salt

Other ingredients include:

B
Ladyfingersvegan(enoughtocoatth
e bottom of your dish)
B Cocoapowderisusedfordusting.

Instructions:

Prepare the Coffee Soaking Liquid as
tOllOWSt

1.  Combinethestrongbrewedcoff
    ee, coffee liqueur (if using),
    and maple
    syrup or agave nectar in a shallow dish.
Combine thoroughly.

2.  Ladyfingers soak: Dip each
    vegan ladyfinger into the coffee

mixture quickly, making sure they are wet but not drenched.

3. Ladyfingers layered: Arrange moistened ladyfingers in the bottom of a serving plate.

4. Individual glasses or a larger dish may be used.

5. To make the cashew cream, follow these steps:

6. Blend the cashews, coconut cream, maple syrup or agave nectar, melted coconut oil, vanilla extract, lemon juice, and a pinch of salt in a blender. Blend till creamy and smooth.

7. Cashew Cream: Distribute half of the cashew cream mixture equally over the layer of wet ladyfingers.

8. Layers should be repeated: On top of the cashew cream, add another layer of
soaked ladyfingers, followed by the remaining cashew cream.

9. Chill: Refrigerate the dish for at least 4 hours, or overnight, to allow the flavors to mingle and the tiramisu to set.

10.   Cocoa powder: Dust the top of the tiramisu with cocoa powder just before
serving.

11.   Serve: Enjoy this plant-based spin on a traditional dessert by serving your
Vegan Tiramisu cold!

This vegan tiramisu is rich and creamy, with all of the same delectable flavors as the traditional version, but without the use of dairy or eggs. It's ideal for special events or as a sweet finish to a meal.

# Donuts with Cinnamon Sugar:

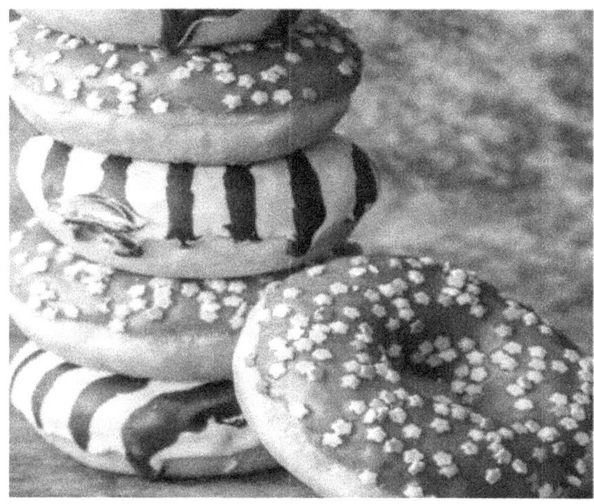

Cinnamon sugar donuts are a traditional and tasty dessert that is simple to make at home. Here's a quick recipe for cinnamon sugar donuts:

Ingredients:

Regarding the Donuts:

B 2cupsregularflour

B

1granulatedsugarcu

p                    B
2tbsp.bakingpowder

B ahalfteaspoonbakingsoda

B 1teaspooncinnamon,1/2teaspoonsalt

B 3/4cupunsweetenedalmondmilk(or
plant-based milk of choice)
B 1/4cupapplesauce,unsweetened

Two tablespoons of melted vegetable or coconut oil

One tsp vanilla essence for the coating of cinnamon sugar:

1/2 cup of sugar, granulated

O   one tsp finely ground cinnamon

O   1/4 cup of heated coconut oil or vegan butter

Guidelines:

1.   Warm up the oven: Turn the oven on to 375°F, or 190°C. Grease a pan for donuts.

2.   Assemble the doughnut batter: Mix the flour, sugar, baking soda, baking powder, salt, and ground cinnamon in a big bowl.

3.   COmbine the applesauce, melted coconut oil, almond milk, and vanilla extract in a another bowl.

4. Mixing until just mixed, pour the wet components into the dry ingredients. Avoid over-mixing.

5. Pour Filling Into Donut Pan: Transfer the batter into a Ziploc bag or piping bag by snipping off the corner.

6. Fill each cavity of the donut pan approximately two thirds full with batter as you pipe it in.

7. Cook: Bake for 10 to 12 minutes, or until the donuts bounce back when lightly touched, in a preheated oven.

8. Tomakesugarcoatingwithcinna mon: For the coating, combine the ground cinnamon and granulated sugar in a shallow basin.

9. Inaanotherbowl,melttheveganbutter.

10. ApplyGlazeontheDonuts:After taking the donuts out of the oven and allowing them to cool somewhat, coat each one evenly by dipping it in

melted butter and then rolling it in the cinnamon sugar mixture.

11.    Serve:lmmediatelyservetheci nnamon sugar donuts for optimal flavor and
texture.

12.    Enjoy: Savor these freshly prepared cinnamon sugar donuts with your

preferred plant-based milk or a cup of coffee!

The addictive cinnamon-sugar flavor of conventional fried donuts is retained in these healthy baked donuts.

## Vegan Berry Crumble:

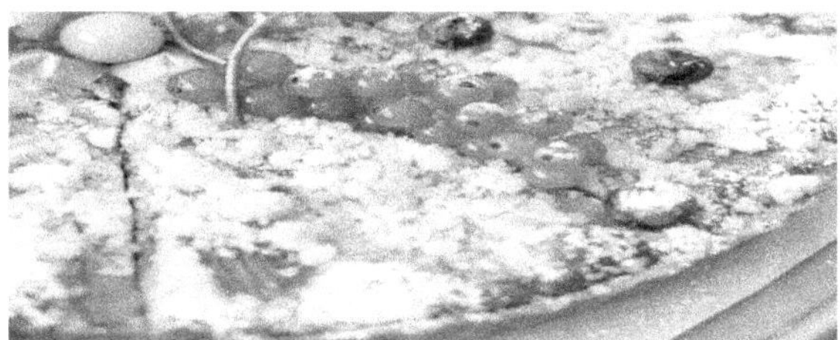

A tasty dessert that highlights the inherent sweetness of berries with a crumbly, delectable topping is vegan berry crumble. This is a basic vegan berry crumble recipe:

Ingredients:

Regarding the Berry Filling:

Four cups of mixed berries, including blackberries, raspberries, blueberries, and strawberries

1/4 cup of sugar, granulated

two tsp cornstarch
One tablespoon of lemon juice
Regarding the Crumble Topper:

One cup of traditional rolled oats Half a cup of almond flour
1/4 cup of chopped nuts, such as pecans, walnuts, or almonds
1/4 cup melted coconut oil
☐ 1/4 cup agave nectar or maple
☐ syrup One tsp vanilla essence
☐ A small amount of salt

Guidelines:

1. Warm up the oven: Set the oven temperature to 350°F

(175°C).

2. Get the berry fillingready:The mixed berries, cornstarch, lemon juice, and granulated sugar should all be combined

in a big basin. Toss until all of the berries have a uniform coating.

3.  Move to the Baking Dish: Spread the berry mixture evenly in a baking dish after transferring it there.

4.  Prepare the Crumble Top: The rolled oats, almond flour, chopped almonds, melted coconut oil, vanilla extract, maple syrup (or agave nectar), and a small amount of salt should all be combined in a different bowl. Stir until all of the ingredients are incorporated.

5.  Crumble While Sipping Berries: Over the berry mixture in the baking dish, evenly distribute the crumble topping.

6.  Cook: Bake for 30 to 35 minutes, or until the crumble topping is golden brown and the berries are bubbling, in a preheated oven.

7. Cool Slightly: Allow the vegan berry crumble to cool for a few minutes before serving.

8. Serve: Serve warm, either on its own or with a scoop of vegan vanilla ice cream or a dollop of coconut whipped cream.

9.    Enjoy: Enjoy your Veg an Berry Crumble as a delicious and fruity dessert!

This vegan berry crumble is a perfect way to enjoy the sweetness of seasonal berries. It's a comforting and wholesome dessert that is sure to be a crowd-pleaser.

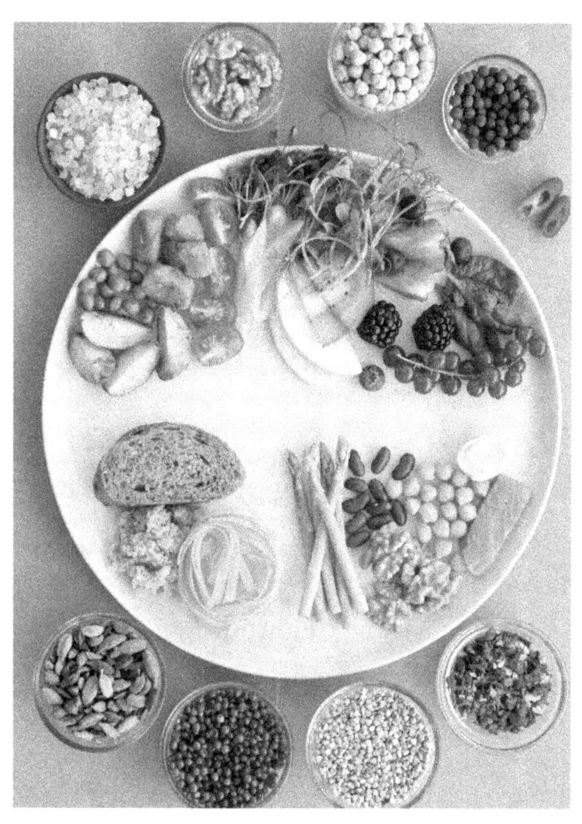

162

# CHAPTER EIGHT

## Tips for Transitioning to a Plant-Based Lifestyle

Transitioning to a plant-based lifestyle can be a rewarding journey for both your health and the environment. Here are some tips to help you make a smooth and sustainable transition:

Educate Yourself:

Learn about the benefits of a plant-based diet and the nutritional needs it fulfills.
Understanding the reasons behind your choice will motivate and empower you.

Take it Gradually:

Instead of making an abrupt change, consider transitioning gradually. Start by incorporating more plant-based meals into your diet and reducing the frequency of animal products.

Explore New Foods:

Experiment with a variety of fruits, vegetables, grains, legumes, nuts, and seeds. Trying new foods will keep your meals interesting and ensure you get a wide range of nutrients.

Meal Planning:

Plan your meals ahead of time to ensure a balanced and satisfying diet. This will help you avoid last-minute decisions that may lead you back to old eating habits.

Find Plant-Based Alternatives:

Investigate plant-based substitutes for your favorite animal items. In grocery shops,
there are many tasty plant-based alternatives to meat, dairy, and other animal-based items.

Home Cooking:

Cooking your own meals gives you more control over the ingredients and guarantees that you eat a diverse range of nutrient- dense foods.

How to Read Labels:

Learn how to read ingredient labels to spot concealed animal products. Dairy, gelatin, and animal-derived additives may be included in some processed foods.

Obtain Help:

Make contact with others who are on a similar path. To share experiences and receive support, join online communities, attend local events, or involve friends and family in your plant-based lifestyle.

Keep Hydrated:

Stay hydrated by drinking plenty of water throughout the day. Water is crucial for general health and might aid in the suppression of cravings.

Pay Attention to Your Body:

Take note of your body's cues. If you are feeling tired or notice any nutrient shortages, seek advice from a licensed dietitian or nutritionist.

Experiment with Different Cooking Styles:

To explore new flavors and textures in plant-based foods, experiment with different cooking styles and techniques such as baking, roasting, steaming, and sautéing.

Maintain a Positive Attitude:

Concentrate on the good features of your plant-based journey. Celebrate modest wins and recognize your beneficial impact on your health and the environment.

Plan a Night Out:

In advance, research plant-based options at restaurants or phone ahead to learn about menu options.
Many restaurants are now offering more plant-based choices.

Supplement Wisely:

Consider taking vitamin B12 supplements or other necessary supplements to ensure you are meeting your nutritional needs. Consult with a healthcare professional for personalized advice.
Remember that everyone's journey is unique, and it's important to find an approach that works best for you. Be patient with yourself, and celebrate the positive changes you make along the way.

# CHAPTER NINE

## Frequently Asked questions

Certainly! Here are some frequently asked questions (FAgs) related to plant-based and dairy-free eating:

1. What is a plant-based diet?

A plant-based diet is centered around whole, plant-derived foods such as fruits, vegetables, grains, legumes, nuts, and seeds. It minimizes or excludes animal products like meat, dairy, and eggs.

2. What is the distinction between vegan and plant-based diets?

While both names suggest a plant-based diet, veganism goes beyond eating to prohibit all animal products, including

those used in lifestyle (e.g., clothing,
cosmetics). Plant- based eating is
largely concerned with
dietary choices.

3. Is a plant-based diet appropriate for people of all ages?

A well-planned plant-based diet can be beneficial to people of all ages, including youngsters and the elderly. It is critical to consume a well-balanced diet and get individualized counsel from a healthcare practitioner.

4. How can I obtain adequate protein on a vegan diet?

Beans, lentils, tofu, tempeh, nuts, seeds, and whole grains are all plant-based protein sources. A variety of these foods consumed throughout the day helps to guarantee appropriate protein consumption.

5. Can a plant-based diet supply all of the needed nutrients?

Yes, a well-balanced plant-based diet can supply all necessary nutrients. However, nutrients such as B12, iron, calcium, and omega-3 fatty acids should be prioritized.

As needed, consider supplements or fortified foods.

6. Are plant-based diets appropriate for athletes?

A plant-based diet can be beneficial to athletes. It is critical to consume enough calories, eat a range of nutrient-dense foods, and pay attention to protein sources. Many top athletes use plant-based diets.

7. How do I substitute dairy in my diet?

Plant-based alternatives to dairy include almond milk, soy milk, coconut milk, and oat milk. There are also nondairy yogurts, cheeses, and ice creams produced from almonds, soy, or coconut.

8. Are there any health benefits to avoiding dairy?

When dairy is removed from the diet, some people report improved digestion, less inflammation, and clearer skin. However, it is critical to substitute dairy minerals such as calcium and vitamin D with alternative sources.

9.	Can I have dessert on a plant- based diet?

Absolutely! Plant-based dessert options abound, including fruit-based delights, vegan cookies, cakes, and ice creams produced with nondairy substitutes.

10.   How do I deal with social situations and eating out while following a plant- based diet?

When dining out, communicate your dietary preferences ahead of time. Many restaurants include plant-based options, and being specific about your requirements can help ensure a satisfying dinner. If necessary,
bring plant-based dishes to social gatherings.

10.   Isitmoreexpensivetofollowapla
nt- based diet?

While some specialty plant-based products can be expensive, a plant-based diet based on whole foods can be cost-effective. Grains, beans, and vegetables are often more affordable than meat and dairy.

11.   Canlloseweightonaplant-b
ased diet?

Many people experience weight loss

on a plant-based diet due to the increased consumption of nutrient-dense, low-calorie foods. However, individual results vary, and portion control is still important.

Remember that individual needs and responses may differ, and consulting with healthcare professionals, nutritionists, or dietitians can provide personalized guidance.

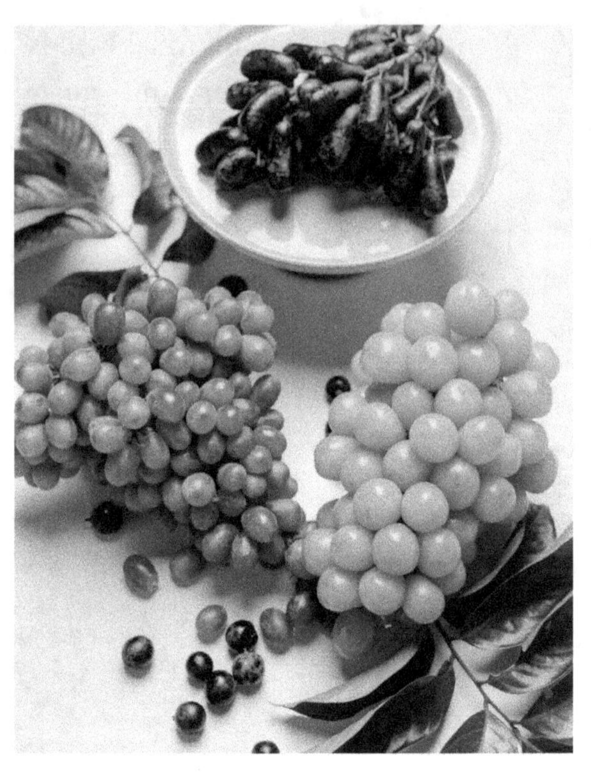

172

# CONCLUSION

In conclusion, embracing a plant-based, dairy-free lifestyle opens the door to a world of flavorful and nutritious culinary possibilities. A plant-based diet not only benefits personal health but also contributes to environmental sustainability and the well- being of animals. The journey toward a
plant-based and dairy-free lifestyle is marked by creativity in the kitchen, as individuals explore the diverse array of fruits, vegetables, grains, legumes, nuts, and seeds. The demand for plant-based cookbooks has grown exponentially, reflecting the increasing interest in this lifestyle.

A plant-based, dairy-free cookbook serves as an invaluable resource, providing a
wealth of recipes that cater to different tastes and dietary preferences. From

vibrant smoothie bowls to hearty main courses and indulgent desserts, these cookbooks offer a myriad of options to satisfy every palate.

The recipes not only focus on replacing animal products but also celebrate the abundance and versatility of plant-derived ingredients.

As more people recognize the positive impact of plant-based eating on their health and the planet, the popularity of plant-based, dairy-free cookbooks continues to rise.

These cookbooks are not just guides to preparing meals; they serve as companions on a journey toward a more conscious and compassionate way of living. By exploring the pages of such cookbooks, individuals can embark on a culinary adventure that not only nourishes the body but also brings joy to the act of preparing and sharing wholesome, plant-based meals.

In the world of plant-based, dairy-free cooking, every dish is an opportunity to celebrate the vibrant colors, flavors, and textures that nature provides. Through thoughtful and innovative recipes, these cookbooks inspire a lifestyle that harmonizes with both personal well-being and the greater environment. As we savor the delightful creations from plant-based,

dairy-free cookbooks, we not only
nourish our bodies but also contribute
to a sustainable and compassionate
way of living for the benefit of
ourselves and future generations.

www.ingramcontent.com/pod-product-compliance
Lightning Source LLC
Chambersburg PA
CBHW070921260726
48661CB00003B/786